Pathology

For Churchill Livingstone

Publisher: Timothy Horne
Project Editor: Barbara Simmons
Copy Editor: Jane Ward
Project Controller: Nancy Arnott
Design Direction: Erik Bigland, Charles Simpson
Indexer: Anne McCarthy
Page Layout: Gerard Heyburn

Churchill's Mastery of Medicine

Pathology

Paul Bass

BSc MD MRCPath
Consultant Histopathologist and Honorary Clinical Teacher
Southampton University Hospitals Trust
Southampton

Clair du Boulay

DM FRCPath
Consultant and Senior Lecturer in Histopathology
Southampton University Hospitals Trust
Southampton

Illustrations by
Peter Lamb

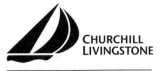

CHURCHILL
LIVINGSTONE

NEW YORK, EDINBURGH, LONDON, MADRID, MELBOURNE,
SAN FRANCISCO AND TOKYO 1997

CHURCHILL LIVINGSTONE
Medical Division of Pearson Professional Limited

Distributed in the United States of America by Churchill
Livingstone Inc., 650 Avenue of the Americas, New York, N.Y.
10011, and by associated companies, branches and
representatives throughout the world.

First published 1997

ISBN 0 443 050031

British Library of Cataloguing in Publication Data
A catalogue record for this book is available from the British
Library.

Library of Congress Cataloging in Publication Data
A catalog record for this book is available from the Library of
Congress.

Medical knowledge is constantly changing. As new information
becomes available, changes in treatment, procedures, equipment
and the use of drugs become necessary. The author and publisher
have, as far as it is possible, taken care to ensure that the
information given in this text is accurate and up to date.
However, readers are strongly advised to confirm that the
information, especially with regard to drug usage, complies with
current legislation and standards of practice.

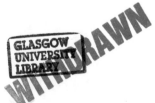

Produced by Longman Singapore Publishers Pte Ltd
Printed in Singapore

The
publisher's
policy is to use
**paper manufactured
from sustainable forests**

*For Frank, Paulina, Aaron, David and Abraham,
without whose forbearance this book would never
have been written.*

Acknowledgements

We would like to thank the following for their helpful comments and for allowing us to adapt some of the pathology material used by Southampton medical students: Professor George Stevenson, Dr David Jones, Dr Bridget Wilkins, Dr Patrick Gallagher, Dr Steve George and Dr Shaoli Zhang.

We are particularly grateful to Dr Susan Burroughs for her detailed comments from the student perspective.

Contents

Using this book

The art of learning

How much do I need to know?

This is a common problem for medical undergraduates. Traditionally, the undergraduate medical curriculum has tended to emphasise factual recall of knowledge, mainly to pass exams. Despite recent changes, curricula are still overloaded with facts. Because of the scientific explosion of knowledge, it is more necessary than ever to be able to sort out what is important and what is less important. There is probably too much emphasis on scientific knowledge and many curricula are unbalanced with little time for learning, communication and interpersonal skills. It could be argued that it is as important to be able to break bad news as to know details about T cell receptors.

All the material in this book is core material. We have eliminated a lot of detail which will be found in larger pathology textbooks. If you know and understand the information in this book, you will have an adequate basis for your ward-based and postgraduate studies. Different students have varying interests and abilities, so that some will inevitably wish to consult larger textbooks and study in more depth than others.

It is essential that you start to develop the skills of deep learning which will form the basis of a lifetime of learning. Qualified doctors learn until they retire. The ability to apply knowledge to clinical situations is fundamental to the diagnostic process. Memorising facts will not enable you to do this. There is no doubt that the majority of medical students find it easier to remember and understand basic science if they can see its relevance. The use of clinical examples and case histories in this book is designed to make the subject more interesting, memorable and understandable. This problem-based approach, combined with integration of subjects (i.e. looking for links between disciplines and subjects) helps understanding. For example, using a clinical case of heart failure helps to understand the mechanisms of oedema and oncotic pressure.

The factors which help people to learn are:

- enjoyment
- relevance
- motivation
- feedback on progress.

General principles of assessment

Most of the assessments or exams which you experience in medical school are of summative type; that is they are designed to pass or fail and to enable you to move on to the next stage of the course. Usually there is little or no feedback on the results.

Formative assessment is a different kind of assessment where the results are used to give feedback to students about their strengths and weaknesses and about their progress.

In this book the self-assessment questions are intended to give you some idea of where there are gaps in your knowledge.

Assessment methods

Multiple choice questions

The multiple choice question (MCQ) is a popular form of assessment in many medical courses. This is because the questions are relatively easy to set and can be marked quickly and efficiently in large numbers by mechanical means. Only very sophisticated MCQs test anything other than factual recall. There is nothing for it but to arm yourself with facts in order to pass an MCQ paper. However, you can use strategies to maximise your marks. For example, if there is a negative marking system, it is not a good idea to guess randomly, but it may be worth making an informed guess in positively marked tests.

Short notes

Short notes questions are designed to test factual knowledge and some elements of reasoning and understanding. The markers usually devise a prototype answer and marks are simply awarded for every item or cluster of items required. No extra points will be given for information which is not strictly relevant. Start your answer with some kind of definition and go on from there. It is a good idea to use simple diagrams wherever possible. You can then refer to them in your explanation.

Essay

The essay gives you the best chance to show how much you understand and can relate one area of knowledge to another. It also tests your ability to organise and present information logically and clearly. It is a communication exercise. Marks may be given not just for factual content but for use of English, presentation (including handwriting) and structure of the essay and how the points and arguments are developed. Use side headings (underlined if necessary) and diagrams. These help to make things clear and will often enable you to communicate your knowledge to the examiner.

Essays are time consuming to mark and may be subject to marker bias and for this reason are often denigrated. However, the skills of essay writing are ones which you must master.

Viva

The viva voce examination can be an alarming experience, but again it is your opportunity to show the examiner not just how much you can recall but your breadth and depth of understanding. The 'viva' is an integral part of most examinations in medicine, both undergraduate and postgraduate. All students find vivas stressful. Sometimes you will feel as though your mind has gone blank when the examiner asks a question. Don't panic; take a deep breath and think for a second or two otherwise you may jump in with the first thing that comes into your head. Try to imagine how you would start the answer if you were writing it down. A simple definition is often a good start. If you do not understand the question then say so, ask for it to be repeated. The viva is a two-way communication process and examiners cannot expect you to give your best if they do not express themselves clearly.

If the question requires an answer listing the causes of a disease, assemble your causes in order of importance. Do not put the most rare one at the top of the list. Common things occur commonly; for example, traumatic crushing of the coronary artery comes very low on the list of causes of myocardial infarction — atheromatous narrowing (furring) of the coronary arteries is by far the most common cause.

If you mention a rare disease, you lay yourself open for the examiner to ask you more about it. This is fine if you know the subject, but not if you don't. Unfortunately, some examiners revel in making candidates uncomfortable and even scoring points off them, although most are more empathic and sympathetic.

Spotter

Usually, the spotter exam is taken in anatomy. However, in more integrated courses, combined anatomy/pathology spotters are becoming common. Usually, there is a series of 'stations' at which there will be a specimen, test result or diagram about which you have to answer questions. You are allowed a certain number of minutes at each station and then you move on to the next one. More sophisticated versions of the spotter may include a clinical case in which you move through a series of stations which all relate to the one case. For example, a pathology pot showing myocardial infarction may be followed by stations with chest X-rays, ECGs or cardiac enzyme results.

Students often feel pressurised during spotter exams and it is a good idea to jot down a precis of the question at a station if you cannot respond, so that if there are a few spare minutes at another, easier station, you can go back to the one which you had trouble with.

Using the self-assessment sections in this book

We have included a mixture of assessment methods for you to use. The answers which we provide will give you some idea where your gaps are and will also help you to organise your answers effectively. Some of the answers contain new material or new examples of basic principles and are designed to build on the basic knowledge in the main text.

We have given factual answers to all the MCQs and answers with discussion points for the case histories.

We have not given comprehensive answers for the essays, short notes questions or viva questions. Where appropriate, we have suggested a way of approaching the question and an outline answer. This is because these questions are designed not just to test factual recall but to show that you can organise, prioritise and apply your knowledge to different situations. In the first chapter of the book, we have outlined the ways of classifying and thinking about diseases which will help you do this.

Pathology, health and disease

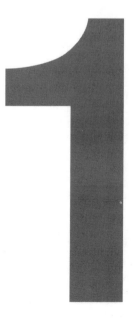

Chapter overview

Pathology is an important discipline which provides the link between basic biological sciences and the practice of medicine. In broad terms, the study of pathology encapsulates the way we think about diseases and about their causes, prevention and classification. Using a more limited definition, pathology is the study of changes which occur in cells and tissues as a result of inborn genetic, extraneous environmental or behavioural damage.

- Pathology is the study of disease processes.
- Epidemiology provides a broad context for understanding pathology.
- Both provide a useful framework for classifying and understanding mechanisms of disease.

1.1 Health, illness and disease

Normal health or well being is a state which most of us experience most of the time. Illness, however, is the subjective state of not feeling well and sickness is a state of social dysfunction, i.e. a role that the individual assumes when ill. There is a wide range of normality and the human body can readily adapt to changes in the environment (e.g. by an increase in haemoglobin at an altitude where oxygen levels are low). Disease or ill health occurs when these limits of normality are overreached.

Disease is defined as a physiological or psychological dysfunction. It can be caused by an obvious structural abnormality such as a broken bone or a tumour or may be less well defined, as in the case of anorexia nervosa. All diseases have certain aspects which can form the basis of a classification and these include:

- epidemiology
- aetiology
- pathogenesis.

Epidemiology

Epidemiology provides a wider context for the study, classification and diagnosis of diseases. Data recorded about incidence, prevalence, morbidity and mortality relate to populations, rather than individuals.

Knowledge of epidemiology is important for:

- providing causal clues
- identifying risk factors and risk markers
- planning and executing disease prevention and health promotion
- providing adequate health care facilities
- setting up population screening programmes
- evaluating health care interventions.

Factors which affect the **incidence** (number of new cases occurring in a defined population over a defined time period) and **prevalence** (number of cases found in a defined population at a stated time) of disease include:

- time: how the disease has varied over the course of time
- place: how the disease varies geographically
- person: what are the personal characteristics of those who suffer from the disease and how they differ from those who do not suffer from the disease, e.g. in age, sex, occupation, race, social class, behaviour.

Changes in the incidence of disease with time may result from preventative measures, such as immunisation programmes, or may reflect changes in social conditions. For example, better housing conditions have led to a decrease in tuberculosis, and increased smoking has led to an increase in heart disease and lung cancer. The drop in the number of cases of tuberculosis antedated BCG immunisation and antibiotics and was mainly a result of better housing and social conditions.

Many diseases show significant geographical variations: in developed countries, heart disease, cancer and psychiatric illnesses are common whereas in underdeveloped countries, malnutrition and infection are often the commonest health problems. Different infectious agents are common in different geographical areas.

There are many well documented associations between disease and occupation:

- coal miners: pneumoconiosis (coal dust disease of the lungs)
- dockyard workers: asbestosis (asbestos-related scarring in the lungs); mesothelioma (malignant tumour of the lung pleura)
- rubber and dye workers: bladder cancer through the effect of chemicals
- hardwood manufacturing: nasal cancer as a result of inhalation of wood dust.

Aetiology (causes of disease)

Diseases result from the interaction between individuals and their environment. Some diseases are the inevitable result of environmental factors (e.g. being run over by a bus) whereas others result from an environmental or behavioural factor acting in conjunction with a genetic predisposition, e.g. smokers with a strong family history of heart disease.

Some examples are:

- genetic: Down's syndrome (extra chromosome 21)
- infective: bacteria, viruses, fungi
- chemical: cirrhosis of the liver caused by alcohol damage; respiratory failure as a result of paraquat poisoning affecting lungs
- radiation: post-irradiation cancer (e.g. skin cancer, squamous cell carcinoma) developing in the skin of a breast irradiated for mammary carcinoma
- mechanical: traumatic crush injury.

Idiopathic disease. In some instances, the underlying cause of a disease is obscure. Many euphemisms are used for this, including idiopathic, cryptogenic, essential and spontaneous. Cause unknown is a simpler and more honest way of saying the same thing.

Pathogenesis (mechanisms of disease)

The pathogenesis of a disease is the mechanism by which the cause(s) interact with the target cells or tissue to produce injury. Cells and tissues are relatively limited in the ways in which they can respond to insult or injury. There are a few fundamental processes which underlie most diseases:

- inflammation: response to injury in living vascularised tissue
- degeneration: deterioration of cell function resulting from metabolic disease or ageing
- carcinogenesis: process of transformation of cells from the normal, controlled to the neoplastic, autonomous state
- immune reactions: specific responses to foreign organisms or material.

Classification of disease

The most useful disease classification is based on the pathogenesis or underlying mechanism. Broadly speaking, diseases can be classified into two categories: 'congenital' or 'acquired'. Congenital diseases are present at birth even though they may not be recognised or recognisable at that time. Acquired diseases only occur after birth. Both congenital and acquired diseases can be classified further (Table 1).

1.2 Ways of thinking about diseases

It is useful to have a logical framework for thinking about diseases. There are several ways of organising information about these, which include:

- definition: clinical or pathological
- epidemiological: incidence, age/gender, geography, race
- clinical presentation: symptoms and signs
- underlying pathology: understanding mechanisms of disease with changes in tissues visible by naked eye (macroscopic), changes seen only down the microscope (microscopic) and tissue function (pathopysiology)
- differential diagnosis: other diseases which may be similar
- treatment and management: drugs, surgery, counselling
- prognosis: natural history of disease, disease outcome.

Diseases are often discussed in terms of their morbidity (degree of 'illness' involved) and mortality. 5- and 10-year survival rates are often used as an expression of the disease outcomes. For example, in some types of lung cancer, the 5-year survival rate is 0%. Relative risk is the incidence in the particular population (e.g. lung cancer in heavy smokers) divided by the incidence in the unexposed or general population.

Table 1 Classification of diseases based on their pathogenesis

Type	Basis	Examples
Congenital	Genetic	Reduction or absence of blood clotting factor VIII leads to haemophilia A (X chromosome linked) Defective epithelial ion transport mechanism causes thick, sticky mucous secretions which leads to cystic fibrosis (autosomal recessive)
	Non-genetic	Intrauterine rubella infection (German measles) leads to deafness/blindness in the fetus
Acquired	Inflammatory	Dermatitis (eczema, inflammation of the skin), rheumatoid disease (inflammation of joints/arthritis)
	Vascular	Atherosclerosis (deposition of lipid with thickening of blood vessels) leading to a cerebrovascular accident (stroke), myocardial infarction (heart attack)
	Growth disorders	Cancer
	Metabolic	Gout (deposition of uric acid crystals in joints and tissues), kidney stones, diabetes mellitus (lack of insulin)
	Degenerative	Alzheimer's disease, Parkinson's disease
	Drug induced	Bone marrow suppression, skin rashes, renal failure
	Infective	Viral, bacterial or fungal diseases

Self-assessment: questions

The principles of health and disease are rarely dealt with in pathology exams. More commonly, knowledge of their definitions and the processes of diagnosis of disease are assumed in more integrated exams (e.g. epidemiology, pathology and physiology).

Multiple choice questions

1. The following statements are correctly paired:
   a. Idiopathic — cause unknown
   b. Pathogenesis — direct cause of disease
   c. Congenital — present at birth
   d. Prognosis — likely disease outcome
   e. Aetiology — mechanism of disease production

2. The following are examples of genetic diseases:
   a. Haemophilia (factor VIII deficiency)
   b. Down's syndrome
   c. Colour blindness
   d. Munchausen's syndrome
   e. Pulmonary asbestosis

3. The following statements are correct:
   a. Malignant mesothelioma is caused by inhalation of coal dust
   b. Tongue cancer is more common in smokers
   c. Human papilloma virus is the cause of cervical cancer
   d. Breast cancer is more common in women who have not had children
   e. Fallot's tetralogy is a form of congenital heart disease

4. The following are correctly paired:
   a. Incidence — number of cases in a population at a given time
   b. Symptoms — features of an illness that the patient notices
   c. Prevalence — number of new cases in a population over a given time
   d. Morbidity — number of deaths in a population
   e. Sensitivity of a screening test — number of patients with the disease who have a positive screening test

Case history

> A 9-year-old boy with cystic fibrosis presents to his local hospital with a chest infection. He has chest pain and is coughing up foul smelling, green sputum.

1. What is cystic fibrosis?

2. What is the pathogenesis of the child's chest infection?

> He is treated with antibiotics and makes a swift recovery.

3. What other problems do patients with cystic fibrosis have and what is the prognosis of the disease?

Essay/short notes

1. What factors may affect the incidence and prevalence of a disease? Illustrate your answer with examples of two contrasting diseases.
2. What is meant by the term 'screening'? What factors influence the success of a screening programme?
3. What factors influence the prognosis of a disease?

Viva questions

1. Define 'congenital'. How does this differ from the term 'genetic'?
2. How do aetiology and pathogenesis differ?
3. What is meant by an acquired disease? What are the main categories of acquired disease?
4. What type of disease may have a high incidence but a low prevalence (and vice versa)?

Self-assessment: answers

Multiple choice answers

1. a. **True.** Idiopathic, essential and primary are all terms used to mean cause unknown.
   b. **False.** Pathogenesis is the mechanism by which the causal agent(s) act upon the body systems to produce the disease.
   c. **True.** The term 'congenital' means that the pathological process has occurred during embryonic development. It is important to remember that the congenital disease/defect may not cause any problems until months or years after birth (e.g. various forms of congenital heart disease).
   d. **True.** The prognosis of a disease is an estimate of its outcome.
   e. **False.** The aetiology of a disease is the causal agent.

2. a. **True.** Haemophilia is an inherited disorder of blood clotting. The genetic defect is linked to the X chromosome and is carried by females and mainly expressed in disease form in males. The gene defect causes a defect in factor VIII production and thus the clotting cascade is interrupted and patients suffer from a bleeding tendency.
   b. **True.** Down's syndrome is the commonest chromosomal disorder and most affected children (95%) have trisomy 21 (i.e. an extra chromosome 21). Their total chromosome count is therefore 47. Two other common trisomies are trisomy 18 (Edward's syndrome) and trisomy 13 (Patau's syndrome).
   c. **True.** Colour blindness is another X-linked genetic disorder, manifesting in males.
   d. **False.** Patients suffering from Munchausen's syndrome have fictitious illnesses with frequent admissions to hospital with repeated investigations and sometimes surgery.
   e. **False.** Asbestosis is a fibrotic lung disease which is acquired from industrial exposure to asbestos dust.

3. a. **False.** Asbestos exposure is the cause of this tumour. The risk of developing malignant mesothelioma is much greater in people exposed to large amounts of asbestos (e.g. dockyard workers) than the normal population. In 90% of people with this cancer, there is evidence of asbestos exposure and there is good experimental evidence that asbestos is a direct causal factor. Interestingly, mesotheliomas can arise from the peritoneum, pericardium and rarely the tunica of the testis.
   b. **True.** Heavy smokers and alcohol drinkers have a ten-fold 'relative risk' of cancers in the oral cavity. Relative risk is the incidence in exposed people, divided by the incidence in unexposed people.
   c. **False.** The statement implies that HPV is *the single causative factor* of cervical cancer. The virus can be found in cervical cancers and pre-cancers, but this does not mean it is the cause. Studies show that other factors such as smoking, nutritional status and immune status interact to produce the tumour.
   d. **True.** One of the factors known to increase the risk of developing breast cancer is the length of time the female breast is exposed to high levels of oestrogen. Therefore, women who have not had children (nulliparous women), or have had an early menarche or late menopause are at risk. It may be that high peaks of oestrogen over a long time period trigger some epithelial cells to become autonomous. This could be by way of oestrogen receptor-linked growth factor production (see Ch. 3, 'Growth factors').
   e. **True.** Fallot's tetralogy is the most common type of cyanotic congenital heart disease.

4. a. **False.** Incidence is the number of new cases in a population over a given time.
   b. **True.** The terms 'symptoms' and 'signs' are often used interchangeably. Signs are the clinical manifestations of a disease which the clinician elicits.
   c. **False.** Prevalence is the number of cases in a population at any one time.
   d. **False.** The term 'morbidity' relates to illness, not death (mortality).
   e. **True.** Screening for disease is an important concept, particularly in cancer prevention. Screening is the process whereby apparently healthy people are investigated in order to detect unrecognised disease. Although 'mass screening' does exist (e.g. all babies are screened for phenylketonuria at birth) most screening targets certain 'at risk' groups. The screening programmes for female breast and cervical cancer target subgroups of the population who are most at risk (i.e. females of certain age groups). Screening involves a cheap diagnostic test, such as a cervical smear or mammogram, which picks up those with early, treatable forms or precursors of the disease. The test must be sensitive enough to pick up all cases, but not oversensitive so that 'false-positive' results occur. In a perfect test, the sensitivity (true positives) and specificity (true negatives) will each be 100%.

Case history answer

1. Cystic fibrosis (CF) is characterised by the production of abnormally sticky mucous secretions

by exocrine glands. This causes blockage of the ducts in organs such as the pancreas, lung and reproductive tissues, leading to failure of function. Susceptibility to lung infections is a particular problem. The diagnosis can be made by the finding of elevated chloride and sodium concentrations in sweat. CF is an autosomal recessive disease. The CF gene has been located on the long arm of chromosome 7 and is known to code for a chloride ion-linked transmembrane regulator protein. There are numerous mutations of the CF gene. The prevalence of carriers of the gene is very high (of the order of 1:25 Caucasians).

2. This case illustrates the relationship between pathogenesis and aetiology. The aetiology or cause of the lung infection will probably be a bacterium such as *Staphylococcus aureus* or *Pseudomonas aeruginosa*. The pathogenesis of the infection is more complex. CF leads to retention of sticky secretions in the lung; these sticky secretions can then be colonised by bacteria, some of which will be pathogenic (disease causing) and flourish, infecting the lung and inciting an inflammatory reaction with pus formation. Intense physiotherapy is needed to help drain the secretions and antibiotic therapy is mandatory.

3. CF patients have numerous systemic problems. Failure of pancreatic function, requiring enzyme supplements and in some patients insulin therapy, and liver and cardiopulmonary failure are the most important. Although the prognosis of CF is improving with better therapeutic regimens and it may ultimately be cured by gene therapy, the disease still causes premature death; very few patients with CF survive beyond the age of 40 years.

Essay/short notes answers

In all these three questions, start off with a definition of the term; for example, prognosis is the outcome of a disease, which relates to its natural history and biological behaviour. If the question is a short answer question then be brief and include the main points which are relevant. It is always a good idea to use a concrete example to illustrate the theory which you are explaining, for example the cervical screening programme.

If the question is to be answered as a full essay, then you can expand the main points and put them in context with your other knowledge, by either using more examples or bringing in other relevant material. Always use a simple essay plan to organise your thoughts and discussion.

1. An essay plan for a discussion of prevalence and incidence of a disease might follow the pattern:

   a. introduction: epidemiology, what it is, why it is important as a background for understanding disease
   b. definitions of incidence and prevalence

   c. what general overall factors affect incidence and prevalence: give examples of the following factors: time, place, person
   d. describe two examples which will illustrate the above points, e.g. choose an inherited disease such as cystic fibrosis and an infectious disease such as influenza or AIDS in contrast
   e. conclusion and summary.

2. The main points to be covered are:

   a. the definition of screening
   b. the relationship between the natural history of a disease and the target population
   c. the acceptability of the screening method
   d. sensitivity and specificity in relation to false-negative and false-positive results
   e. examples, e.g. cervical screening.

3. The prognosis of a disease will vary for each patient and depends upon:

   a. the nature of the disease
   b. how long the patient has had the disease
   c. the general state of health of the patient: the presence of other diseases, and nutritional status
   d. the age of the patient
   e. the response of the patient to the treatment available.

There are many examples of changing prognosis related to factors of an individual patient's status, e.g. *Candida* fungal infection in a healthy individual is a minor illness, whereas in an HIV-infected patient it may be fatal; influenza in a healthy 20-year-old is a self-limiting illness, whereas in an elderly bed-ridden patient, it may lead to pneumonia and death.

Viva answers

Use the same approach to answering the viva questions. It is a good idea to start off with a definition of the subject or topic and then give examples in the same way as for a short answer question. However, the examiners often ask questions which may deflect you from a logical sequence, because they will be looking for depth and breadth of knowledge. You will have to keep prioritising and re-organising your knowledge as you go along.

1. Congenital disease is present at birth, but not necessarily inherited. Genetic disease is inherited but will not necessarily manifest at birth. For example, rubella infection is congenital whereas haemophilia is a genetic disorder.

2. Aetiology is the cause of a disease whereas pathogenesis is the underlying process that gives rise to the disorder. For example:

   • aetiology: mycobacterium tuberculosis organisms cause tuberculosis

- pathogenesis: delayed hypersensitivity response (T cells and macrophages) to the organism gives rise to the destructive granulomas that characterise the disease.

3. An acquired disease is one that occurs after birth as a result of exposure to the causative environmental factors, for example infections, occupational exposure (asbestos) and autoimmune disease. The main categories are given in Table 1.

4. Incidence is the number of cases occurring in a defined population over a stated period of time whereas prevalence is the number of cases in a defined population at a given time; for example, influenza, cystic fibrosis.

The diagnostic process: from clinical reasoning to molecular biology

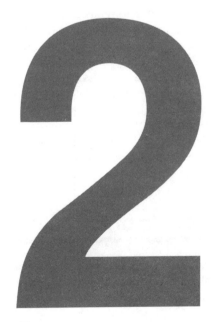

Chapter overview

Patients present with symptoms and a clinical examination elicits signs which suggest a diagnosis. Examination of specimens (blood, urine, faeces, tissue samples) in the various pathology laboratories helps confirm this diagnosis and monitor treatment.

- Diagnosis involves clinical skills and laboratory tests.
- Specialist pathological techniques can aid in diagnosis.
- Special stains, immunohistochemistry and molecular techniques are now routinely used.

2.1 **Diagnosis**

Diagnosis is the act of identifying a disease in an individual patient and is based on clinical history, physical examination and investigation. An understanding of and ability to integrate a knowledge of the classification, epidemiology and mechanisms of disease processes are essential. Making a diagnosis involves:

- taking a clinical history of symptoms: what the patient has noticed is wrong (e.g. cough, breathlessness, pain)
- clinical examination for signs: what the doctor finds wrong on examination (e.g. lumps, rashes, abnormal lung sounds).

The clinician then works through a series of questions:

- which organ system is most likely to be affected?
- which category of disease do the signs and symptoms most likely suggest, e.g. inflammation, malignancy or poisoning?
- do other factors such as race, age, sex, behavioural patterns or occupation of the patient provide clues to the diagnosis?

The diagnostic process involves testing a series of hypotheses based upon the clinician's knowledge of the frequency of occurrence of the symptoms and signs in different disease states and upon the probability of these occurring in the population from which the patient is drawn. A list of possible diagnoses is constructed, known as the differential diagnosis, beginning with the most likely disease and progressing to include diagnoses which are less likely but are important to exclude. Reaching a diagnosis enables the clinician to start treatment and to give the patient some idea of the outcome of the disease (prognosis).

2.2 **The role of the pathologist**

The pathologist can help the clinician to make a diagnosis by looking at samples of tissue (biopsies) and by using a range of specialised laboratory techniques to refine the differential diagnosis. It is important to remember that pathology includes a large number of sub-specialities. Each of these investigates disease processes by examining or studying different body samples. For example, haematologists are concerned with disorders of the blood, whilst immunologists are concerned with disorders of the body's immune system. The clinical diagnosis can often only be made after several samples of blood, urine and tissue have been examined and the results assessed in the light of the patient's history and the clinical findings.

Histology

Basic histological techniques involve the fixation and processing of biopsied or excised tissues so that they can be finely sliced to a thickness of no more than 4–5 microns (μm) and stained on a glass slide to be looked at under the light microscope. Cells can be scraped or aspirated from various parts of the body and placed directly on glass slides and stained; this is called cytology. In these preparations, abnormal cell morphology can be identified. Sometimes, clinicans require a very urgent diagnosis during surgery and small amounts of tissue can be quickly frozen, sectioned and looked at within a few minutes ('frozen sections').

It is also possible to look at tissues at a much higher magnification using the electron microscope. This is an expensive and specialised technique, not used routinely, but it enables us to see cell structures to the level of individual mitochondria, nuclei and smaller. This is known as ultrastructural examination. Viral particles in cells can be seen by electron microscopy.

The autopsy

Pathologists also perform autopsies, i.e. the examination of the body after death. The main purpose of the autopsy is to determine the cause of death, but the pathologist can also confirm a clinical diagnosis made in life, as well as identifying diseases or conditions which were not apparent in life. Discussions between clinicians and pathologists about autopsy findings often lead to new insights into the causes and outcomes of disease. Autopsies provide useful material for teaching, and the 'post-mortem demonstration' is a popular format in which students can see and discuss at first hand the pathological processes in disease.

Special stains

Histopathologists investigate disease processes by examining tissue specimens and use a routine haematoxylin and eosin (H & E) stain to look at the tissue on slides. You will see examples of this stain in pathology or histology practical classes. However, there is a range of stains which can be used to highlight specific types of tissue and cell product. Some of these are highly specialised and used rarely, others will commonly be used in pathology (Table 2).

Table 2 Examples of stains used for specific diagnostic purposes

Stain	Diagnostic use
Reticulin (Retic)	Delineates fibrous connective tissue: important in the diagnosis of lung or liver fibrosis (cirrhosis)
Periodic acid Schiff (PAS)	Stains for mucin and aids the diagnosis of mucin-producing (PAS+) cancer
Ziehl Nielsen (ZN)	Stains acid- and alcohol-fast bacilli in tissues, which is diagnostic for mycobacterial infection

Immunohistochemistry

This technique provides the pathologist with a powerful tool for demonstrating and identifying proteins, glycolipids and carbohydrates, which may be normal tissue constituents or produced as a result of a pathological process. Immunohistochemistry is based on the specificity of antibody–antigen binding. Monoclonal antibodies (antibodies having only one antigenic target) or polyclonal antibodies (a group of antibodies having a range of antigens) can be made against a range of human antigens (Fig. 1 and Ch. 7). They can be applied to human tissue sections or cytology preparations and will bind wherever their antigen is present. The antibody can be tagged with an enzyme that catalyses a colour reaction or a fluorescent dye so that the antibody and, by implication, the antigen can be visualised (a simple example is given in Fig. 2). Immunohistochemistry has enabled pathologists to learn much about the distribution of tissue antigens in both health and disease and has increased the accuracy of diagnosis. Figure 2 shows the principles of an immunoperoxidase technique of staining tissues.

Unfortunately, the routine immunohistochemical techniques only detect antigens; they give no information about whether the tissue itself is producing the

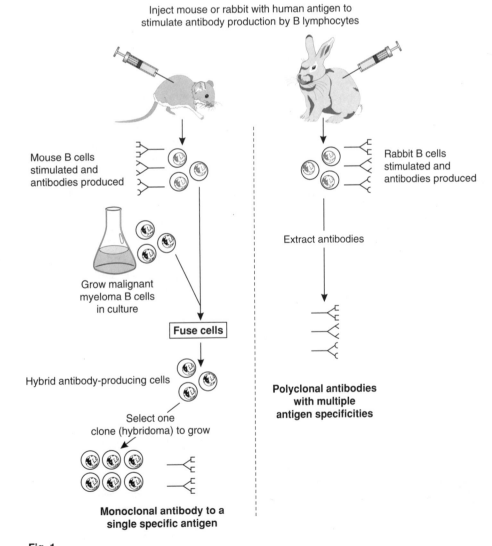

Inject mouse or rabbit with human antigen to stimulate antibody production by B lymphocytes

Mouse B cells stimulated and antibodies produced

Rabbit B cells stimulated and antibodies produced

Grow malignant myeloma B cells in culture

Extract antibodies

Fuse cells

Hybrid antibody-producing cells

Polyclonal antibodies with multiple antigen specificities

Select one clone (hybridoma) to grow

Monoclonal antibody to a single specific antigen

Fig. 1
Monoclonal and polyclonal antibody production.

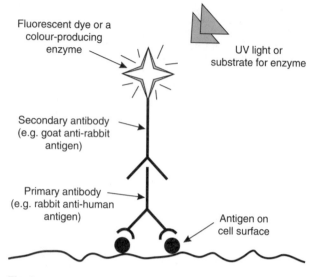

Fig. 2
Diagram of the basic immunohistochemical techniques to visualise antigens.

Principles of hybridisation
• DNA is double stranded • Bonds between complementary bases hold strands together (**Cytosine** ◄─► **Guanine**; **Adenine** ◄─► **Thymine**) • Heat/alkalinise DNA — separation of strands ('denaturation') occurs • Cool separated strands — *complementary* double strands re-form • Labelled complementary single-strand DNA can identify a DNA sequence (e.g. a gene) in intact cells or disrupted cell preparations

antigen, i.e. has switched on the appropriate genetic apparatus to make it. The cells in the tissue may, for instance, have taken up protein from the surrounding tissue fluid. Examples of diagnostic immunohistochemistry are given in Table 3.

Molecular biology techniques

New techniques for looking at chromosomes, genes, DNA, RNA and proteins are being developed continuously. Although many of these techniques are currently used in research, there is no doubt that some have and will become routine clinical tests.

Details of the individual techniques are beyond the scope of this book. A good understanding of the structure of DNA and knowledge of the 'DNA–RNA–protein' pathway will help to understand the principles of molecular biology (Fig. 3).

In situ hybridisation
Molecular techniques can be used to probe the gene and determine whether specific DNA sequences or mRNA

molecules are present and being used. The probes must have a complementary sequence to the DNA or mRNA under study (see the box above). They can then be labelled with either a radioisotope or a non-radioactive enzyme system and applied to a tissue section. Under the correct conditions the probe will 'hybridise' with and identify its complementary nucleic acid sequence in the tissue. The probe can then be visualised and the location, number or type of cell containing the DNA/RNA can be seen down the microscope. The use of fluorescent labels for in situ hybridisation (known as FISH) has increased the usefulness of this technique, for example in characterising chromosomal rearrangements such as microdeletions in genetic and malignant disorders.

Dot blot analysis
This technique does not look for DNA/RNA in tissue slides; rather DNA/RNA is extracted from the tissues, which are, therefore, destroyed. The extracts can then be 'dotted' onto a membrane and the target sequence can then be detected by hybridisation with a specific probe. The product, a 'dot blot', can be used to give an idea of the amount of target DNA/RNA in the tissue: the more intense the dot the more nucleic acid present.

Southern, Northern and Western blot analysis
These techniques are named as directional puns after Edward Southern who invented the first method for examining DNA. In these techniques, DNA fragments

Table 3 Examples of diagnostic immunohistochemistry

Antibody	Diagnostic use
Immunoglobulin	Identification of immunoglobulin-bearing or immunoglobulin-producing cells (e.g. plasma cells) or the deposition of immunoglobulin in tissues (e.g. renal glomerulus); can help to confirm the diagnosis of malignant lymphoma (neoplastic proliferations of cells of the lymphoid system) and glomerulonephritis
Cytokeratin (a filamentous protein present in epithelial cells)	The expression of cytokeratin by a tumour may help differentiate between an epithelial and a non-epithelial origin
Neural proteins	Some of these are very specific for the diagnosis of neural/glial tumours e.g. glial fibrillary acidic protein (GFAP)

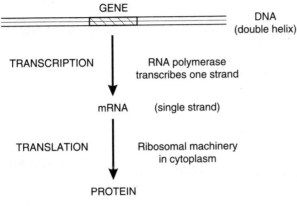

Fig. 3
DNA–RNA–protein pathway.

(Southern blotting), mRNA fragments (Northern) or polypeptides (Western) are placed on an electrophoretic gel. The nucleic acid fragments or peptides then migrate through the gel according to their molecular size and are separated as bands which are subsequently blotted onto nylon membranes and either hybridised with specific nucleic acid probes (Southern/Northern) or visualised by labelled antibodies against the peptides (Western).

The polymerase chain reaction (PCR)

This relatively simple technique is now widely used in molecular biology. It allows analysis of DNA or RNA from virtually any tissue specimen. Central to PCR is a chain reaction which amplifies the length of DNA under examination many million fold. This increases the amount of the sequence to be identified to a level that can be easily detected in the laboratory. The sensitivity of the technique is such that the DNA from a single cell can be amplified. The three vital ingredients of the reaction are:

1. The RNA/DNA to be examined (RNA needs to be converted into DNA by reverse transcription)
2. Two oligonucleotides with sequences matching short DNA sequences flanking the DNA fragment of interest: these give the amplification its specificity
3. A heat-soluble DNA polymerase from the pneumophilic organism *Thermus aquaticus*, which can withstand heating and synthesises DNA at high temperatures.

The mixture is heated, dissociating the double-stranded DNA and allowing the single strands to bind to the oligonucleotides. These oligonucleotides then act as primers for the polymerase and a new double-stranded DNA molecule is formed. Twice as much double-stranded DNA is then present and the cycle can be repeated. At the end of several cycles, there will be large amounts of DNA for analysis. The reaction has numerous applications:

- detection of known genetic diseases, e.g. cystic fibrosis
- cross-matching tissues for transplantation (HLA subtyping)
- detecting DNA from microbial infections where there are either too few microbes for visualisation, or too long an identification process
- detection of viral particles
- detecting abnormal genes linked with cancer.

Self-assessment: questions

Multiple choice questions

1. The following are correctly paired:
   a. Tiredness — clinical sign
   b. Prognosis — how the patient's disease will behave
   c. Tuberculosis — PAS stain
   d. Biopsy — autopsy procedure
   e. High blood pressure — clinical sign

2. The following statements are correct:
   a. The immunoperoxidase technique demonstrates cellular production of antigens in tissues
   b. Western blotting techniques are used to analyse DNA
   c. Squamous cell carcinoma may produce cytokeratin intermediate filaments
   d. Frozen sections are a rapid diagnostic technique which can be used intraoperatively
   e. In situ hybridisation techniques can be used to examine RNA in tissues

Case history

A 73-year-old man has smoked 30 cigarettes a day for over 50 years and develops severe, band-like chest pain and breathlessness whenever he exerts himself climbing stairs or walking up a hill. The pain is associated with sweating and nausea. He goes to his GP who notices that the man has cold hands, a weak irregular pulse and abnormal heart sounds.

1. List the symptoms and signs in this case.
2. Why might the patient have these problems?
3. Is the disease process likely to be congenital or acquired?

Short notes

Write short notes on the following:
1. the difference between a symptom and a sign
2. the principle of the PCR reaction; how may it be used in diagnostic practice?

Viva questions

1. Discuss the role of the autopsy in modern medicine.
2. When might electron microscopic examination of tissues be of use?
3. What are the basic principles behind molecular biological techniques?

Self-assessment: answers

Multiple choice answers

1. a. **False.** Tiredness is a symptom which is noticed by the patient. The clinician may be able to elicit a clinical history or signs which will suggest a reason for the tiredness, e.g. anaemia, depression.
   b. **True.** Prognosis is the term used for predicting the outcome of a disease. By understanding the basic mechanisms and processes of disease, it is possible to inform patients about their likelihood of survival or their expected quality of life.
   c. **False.** Tuberculosis is caused by *Mycobacterium tuberculosis*, an acid-fast bacillus which stains positively with the ZN stain. The PAS stain will show the presence of glycogen or mucin in tissue sections.
   d. **False.** A biopsy is a tissue sample which is surgically removed from a living patient to aid in diagnosis of disease. An autopsy is a post-mortem examination made by the pathologist. Autopsies have an important diagnostic role and are also important for teaching and learning more about disease processes.
   e. **True.** High blood pressure (hypertension) is a clinical sign. Most patients will not know whether or not their blood pressure is normal unless it is measured. However, patients may have symptoms suggestive of high blood pressure such as headache.

2. a. **False.** The immunoperoxidase technique demonstrates the *presence* of antigen in tissue sections. Although antigens may have been produced by the cells in which they are visualised, they may have been taken up non-specifically from surrounding structures or extracellular fluids.
   b. **False.** Western blot analysis is used for identification of peptides/proteins.
   c. **True.** Many cancers produce excessive quantities of certain cell products, which can be identified using histochemical or immunohistochemical techniques. For example, a malignant melanoma, a tumour of the pigment-containing cells of the epidermis (melanocytes), may produce excessive melanin which can be seen in diagnostic sections using a special silver stain (Masson Fontana) or by immunostaining for S-100, a calcium-binding protein found in melanocytes. Similarly, squamous cancers produce cytokeratins ('keratins'). Cytokeratins are water-insoluble proteins found in most epithelial cells. These proteins are therefore good markers of epithelial differentiation in tumours.

   d. **True.** The rapid frozen section is used by surgeons who require urgent confirmation of a diagnosis during surgery. They may alter their surgical procedure on this basis (e.g. knowing whether a tumour is benign or malignant may drastically alter the type of operation performed). Surgeons also may ask the pathologists to perform frozen sections on tissue resection margins during cancer operations, to ensure complete removal.
   e. **True.** In situ hybridisation is a very useful technique which enables us to visualise specific DNA sequences or RNA molecules in tissue sections. It has been used to identify viral or bacterial RNA/DNA in tissue sections. Examples include the Epstein–Barr virus in malignant lymphoid tumours and human papilloma virus sequences in cervical cancer and pre-cancer. It has many applications.

Case history answer

1. The patient's symptoms are breathlessness, sweating and nausea on exertion. The signs of his illness elicited by the GP are cold hands, abnormal pulse and heart sounds.
2. This is a very common clinical scenario in the Western world. Many of the symptoms and signs are caused by atherosclerosis (furring of the arteries caused by a lipid-rich deposit in the vessel wall, see p. 48). This pathological process tends to reduce the calibre of vessels supplying the heart, thus compromising its function, particularly when the heart is stressed by the increased demands of exercise.
3. As in many diseases, both genetic and acquired processes have a role to play in the development of atherosclerosis. Inherited abnormalities of lipid metabolism lead to atherosclerosis during childhood, with early death from heart attacks and stroke. Many of the risk factors for atherosclerosis are acquired and can be controlled by alterations to life style. Cigarette smoking is strongly associated with atherosclerosis.

Short notes answers

1. First define the terms 'symptom' and 'sign'. Then give examples: a symptom is what the patient experiences, such as breathlessness, pain, dizziness. A sign is what the clinician can elicit or demonstrate, e.g. a nerve palsy (paralysis), high blood pressure, cyanosis (blue colouring of the skin caused by hypoxia).

2. Define the PCR reaction as a technique which allows analysis of DNA or RNA in most tissues. The underlying principle is that PCR can amplify the amounts of DNA or RNA in the tissue which otherwise might be too small to detect. Examples of its use are to identify viruses, abnormal cancer genes and abnormal inherited disease genes, such as those involved in muscular dystrophy or cystic fibrosis.

Viva answers

1. Although autopsy is felt by some clinicians to be 'redundant' since the advent of modern imaging techniques (e.g. CT and MRI scans), it is still a very important final audit procedure. It:

- correlates clinical findings with pathological processes
- identifies organs involved in 'new' diseases (e.g. HIV)
- is important in teaching and research.

2. Electron microscopy is still very important in identifying viruses. It is also useful in categorising renal glomerular disease processes and can be extremely valuable in identifying intracellular structures or cell connections, which can allow a tumour to be correctly classified (and possibly alter treatment).

Cell growth and adaptation

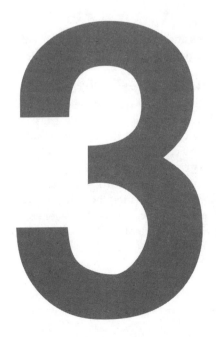

Chapter overview

In order to function appropriately, cells and tissues need to maintain a steady state (homeostasis). Within defined limits, all cells are capable of adapting to a variety of stimuli which may upset normality. Cellular adaptation is the state between a normal unstressed cell and the overstressed injured cell. By definition, an adaptive process is one which is reversible. This chapter covers:

- normal cell growth and the cell cycle
- reversible adaptive responses.

3.1 Normal cell growth

Normal tissue growth depends on a balance between the number of cells actively dividing and the number of cells dying. Labile tissues contain a high proportion of stem cells, which divide frequently and often give rise to cells with a short life span (high cell turnover). In contrast, stable and permanent tissues contain cells which divide only infrequently or not at all and have a longer life span. The three cell types respond differently to stress or injury.

Labile cells. These cells proliferate continuously, have a short life span and a high regenerative capacity. Examples of labile cells include bone marrow 'stem' cells, the epidermal cells of the skin and the gut epithelium.

Stable cells. These divide infrequently but can regenerate when cells are lost. Examples of stable cells include those of liver (hepatocytes) and bone (osteoblasts).

Permanent cells. These divide only in fetal life and cannot be replaced when lost. Instead repair occurs when dead cells are removed and matrix (collagen) fills the gaps. Examples of permanent cells are neurones and cardiac/skeletal muscle cells.

Regeneration

Many tissues and organs contain mixtures of labile, stable and permanent cells. For example, the brain contains neurones, which are permanent cells, and astrocytes, which are stable cells. The ability of cells to divide is intimately linked with the reaction of tissues to injury. Therefore, labile and stable cells can quickly replace dead cells within their population by cell division and replacement with cells of exactly the same type. This is called regeneration (Fig. 4). For example, removal of part of the liver triggers hepatocytes close to the area removed to enter the cell cycle, divide and replace the lost tissue. Successful regeneration of cell populations is dependent on an intact connective tissue matrix around the cells.

Repair

Permanent cells by definition cannot divide and are not able to replace lost cells by the same cell type. Instead repair occurs (Fig. 4). In this process, dead tissue is removed and scar tissue (collagen) fills up the defect. This provides continuity and strength to the tissue but involves loss of the original specialised cell function.

The cell cycle

The four main stages of the cell cycle (Fig. 5) are:

M phase: mitosis when the cell divides (about 1 hour)
G_1 phase: gap 1, the preparation for S phase
S phase: DNA synthesis
G_2 phase: gap 2, during which assembly of the apparatus for the distribution of chromsomes occurs.

In addition, a G_0 phase of the cell cycle is recognised. This phase is non-proliferative and is known as growth arrest.

Permanent cells may enter G_0 phase and stay there, with no further potential for division, and are then said to have undergone terminal differentiation. Other cells in G_0, however, may re-enter the cell cycle at G_1, thereby regaining the proliferative state. This re-entry is stimulated by locally active small-molecular-weight proteins called growth factors.

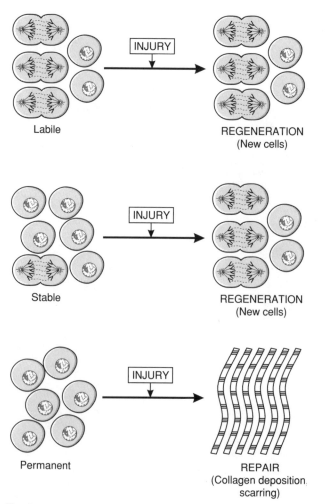

Fig. 4
Regeneration and repair response to injury.

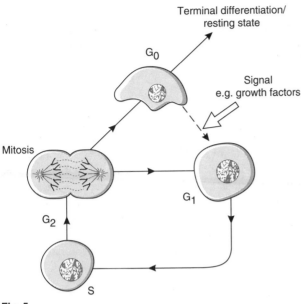

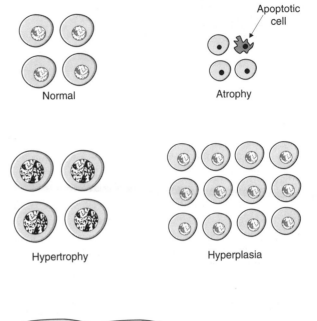

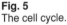

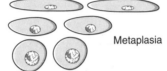

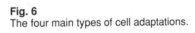

Fig. 5
The cell cycle.

Control of the cell cycle

Growth factors

These are <u>low-molecular-weight proteins</u> which have a similar mechanism of action to hormones. In general, the growth factor is produced by a cell, for example a macrophage, and acts either on the cell itself (autocrine action) or on a neighbouring cell (paracrine action) by linking to cell surface receptors. This interaction activates the receptor and triggers a series of cytoplasmic events usually involving phosphorylation–dephosphorylation of proteins. Ultimately, a signal reaches the nucleus where genes are switched on, new proteins produced and cell growth and division is initiated. Growth factors are thought to be particularly important in stimulating stable, non-proliferating (G_0) cells to enter the cell cycle at G_1 and undergo mitosis.

Cyclins

The cyclins are a family of proteins which seem to coordinate the journey of cells through the different phases of the cell cycle. They form complexes with a protein kinase (phosphorylating) enzyme. The cellular concentration and activity of different cyclins varies through the cycle.

3.2 Cellular adaptation

The normal growth and development of cells is under complex genetic and environmental control. Cellular adaptations, such as atrophy, hypertrophy and some types of hyperplasia remain controlled by <u>normal mechanisms</u> and are reversible.

There are <u>four main adaptive states</u> (Fig. 6):

- atrophy: shrinkage of an organ as a result of decreased cell size (and cell number)

Fig. 6
The four main types of cell adaptations.

- hypertrophy: enlargement of an organ as a result of increased cell size
- hyperplasia: enlargement of an organ through an increase in cell number
- metaplasia: the replacement of one differentiated cell type by another in a tissue or organ.

Atrophy

Atrophy is defined as the shrinkage of a cell by loss of cell substance, which leads to a reduction in size of the whole organ. The cell retreats to a smaller size at which survival is still possible and sequesters its internal structures. In many cases of atrophy, individual cells may undergo apoptosis (programmed cell death, see p. 31).

Physiological causes of atrophy:
- reduction/loss of endocrine stimulation, e.g. shrinkage of testes and ovaries with age.

Pathological causes of atrophy:
- denervation, e.g. wasting of muscle caused by a lack of nerve stimulation, for example in poliomyelitis
- reduced blood supply, e.g. shrinkage of brain caused by furring (atherosclerosis) of carotid arteries
- inadequate nutrition, e.g. wasting of muscles and major organs in starvation
- decreased workload (disuse), e.g. wasting of muscles and bone (osteoporosis) after immobilisation of a bone fracture in a plaster cast.

✳ **Cell structural components are reduced in atrophy**:
- less mitochondria
- less endoplasmic reticulum
- fewer myofilaments.

✳ **The metabolic rate is reduced**:
- less amino acid uptake
- less oxygen consumption
- less protein synthesis.

In atrophy, there is an increase in the number of autophagic vacuoles (intracellular dustbins) which contain fragments of intracellular debris awaiting destruction. Lipofuscin granules are yellow/brown in colour and represent non-digestible fragments of lipids and phospholipids combined with protein within autophagic vacuoles. They are commonly seen in ageing liver and myocardial cells.

Hypertrophy

Bodybuilders and athletes provide the best example of hypertrophy: muscle hypertrophy in response to increased workload. Individual cells increase in size as a result of an increase in their structural components leading to an overall increase in the size of the organ. Protein synthesis increases and its effect is enhanced by a decrease in protein degradation. Hypertrophy is mainly seen in cells which have no capacity for mitotic division, e.g. cardiac and skeletal muscle cells (permanent cells). The limiting factor for the eventual muscle size is the nutrient and blood supply available for oxidative phosphorylation.

Physiological causes of hypertrophy:
- increased workload, e.g. the bodybuilder's skeletal muscle
- hormone stimulation, e.g. the pregnant uterus (smooth muscle hypertrophy).

Pathological causes of hypertrophy:
- increased resistance, e.g. cardiac muscle hypertrophy as a result of working against an increased peripheral resistance in hypertension (high blood pressure)
- physical obstruction, e.g. bladder smooth muscle hypertrophy in outflow obstruction caused by an enlarged prostate gland.

Muscle cells

Hypertrophic muscle cells show:

- increased membrane synthesis
- increased amounts of ATP
- increased enzyme activity
- increased myofilaments.

Endoplasmic reticulum

Hypertrophy of smooth endoplasmic reticulum, i.e. hypertrophy at the subcellular level, can also occur. Drugs such as phenobarbitone cause an increase in the activity of the mixed function oxidase system of liver cells, which results in increased metabolism of other agents. In some instances, this is therapeutically beneficial, in others it can lead to poisoning of the liver cells by toxic metabolites.

Hyperplasia

Enlarged, hyperplastic tissues or organs show an increase in the number of their constituent cells. Tissues such as skin, gut epithelium and bone marrow normally have a high rate of cell turnover and are, therefore, the common sites for hyperplastic growth. Cardiac and skeletal muscle and neurones cannot undergo hyperplasia because they are permanent cells and cannot enter the cell cycle. Endocrine organs often undergo hyperplasia in response to excessive hormonal stimulation.

Physiological causes of hyperplasia:
- hormonal, e.g. the female breast at puberty, the pregnant uterus and the proliferative endometrium in the first half of the menstrual cycle
- cell loss, e.g. regeneration of the liver after partial hepatectomy and regeneration of squamous epithelium in superficial skin wound healing.

Pathological causes of hyperplasia:
- hormonal, e.g. the endometrium in post-menopausal women taking oestrogen-only hormone replacement therapy
- cell destruction, e.g. in ulcerative colitis the colonic mucosa undergoes repeated ulceration (destruction), regeneration and hyperplasia.

Pathological hyperplasia usually occurs in tissues which are exposed to inappropriate hormonal stimulation or to repeated episodes of inflammation, destruction and regeneration. It may progress to uncontrolled cell growth (neoplasia), or it may remain a reversible phenomenon. Since most tissues contain labile and stable and permanent cells, hyperplasia without hypertrophy is uncommon.

Metaplasia

This is usually seen in epithelial tissues and is a reversible change in which one differentiated, adult cell type is replaced by another. The most common type of metaplasia is the replacement of glandular or transitional epithelium by simpler and more robust squamous epithelium. Examples of this are: _with goblet cells_

- bronchial (pseudo-stratified, ciliated columnar) epithelium changes to squamous epithelium in smokers
- transitional bladder epithelium changes to squamous epithelium in people with bladder stones and infection.

Metaplasia probably occurs at the level of the stem cell, which differentiates into the new type of epithelium. Metaplasia is often seen next to neoplastic epithelium, indicating that although this adaptive response is potentially reversible, continued insult to the cells may cause uncontrolled growth and the development of cancer.

Self-assessment: questions

Multiple choice questions

1. The following are correctly paired:
   a. Hepatocytes — permanent cells
   b. Cardiac muscle damage — regeneration
   c. G_0 phase — labile cells
   d. Renal epithelial cells — stable cells
   e. Hyperplasia — permanent cells

2. The following statements are correct:
   a. Bodybuilders can build up muscle indefinitely on a high-protein diet
   b. Smokers' bronchial epithelium is usually atrophic
   c. The lactating breast shows epithelial hyperplasia
   d. Oestrogen-producing ovarian cancer can cause endometrial hyperplasia
   e. The regenerative capacity of the liver is due to the fact that liver cells are labile

3. The following statements are correct:
   a. Atrophy involves necrosis of cells
   b. Metaplasia inevitably leads to neoplasia
   c. Growth factors may inhibit cell growth or division
   d. The myocardium of a hypertensive patient contains more myocardial cells than is normal
   e. The G_1, S and G_2 phases of the cell cycle together make up the interphase

Case histories

Case history 1

A 4-year-old boy is treated for leukaemia (uncontrolled, neoplastic proliferation of bone marrow white cells) with cytotoxic drugs which block the cell cycle and destroy the leukaemic cells. Unfortunately, these drugs also affect the normally rapidly dividing cells of the body.

1. Which of the three cell types in the body (labile, stable or permanent) are most likely to be affected by the treatment?
2. What symptoms and signs may the cytotoxic drugs cause in this patient?
3. Why are these cell cycle-blocking drugs usually given in episodic doses (pulses) with a drug-free interval between treatments?

Case history 2

A 79-year-old woman falls over at home, injuring her left hip. She is taken to hospital and found on clinical examination and X-ray to have fractured the neck of her left femur. Her bones appear less dense than normal on the radiograph and the radiologist suspects osteoporosis. She is otherwise reasonably fit and well for her age and so she is operated on and the fracture fixed with internal screws and a plate. Post-operatively, she makes a good recovery but is rather slow to mobilise. She requires extensive physiotherapy but eventually is able to go home, walking with the aid of a stick.

1. What are the main risk factors for osteoporosis?
2. Why is it important for her to become mobile as quickly as possible post-operatively?

Short notes

Write short notes, giving examples, on the following:

1. Compare and contrast hyperplasia and hypertrophy; how would the tissues return to normal after the stimulus is removed? What factors limit the extent to which hypertrophy can develop?
2. The mechanisms by which a tissue becomes atrophic.

Viva questions

1. Define atrophy, hypertrophy and hyperplasia.
2. Describe the cell cycle; comment on control mechanisms.
3. Compare and contrast regeneration and repair.
4. Describe labile, stable and permanent cells, with examples, and their relationship with the cell cycle.

Self-assessment: answers

Multiple choice answers

1. a. **False.** Hepatocytes are stable cells. Therefore, they can enter the cell cycle and divide in order to replace lost cell numbers.
   b. **False.** Cardiac muscle cells are permanent cells (terminally differentiated) which do not enter the cell cycle. Death of cardiac muscle cells, which occurs in myocardial infarction, leads to replacement by scar tissue (collagen). This process is known as repair.
   c. **False.** In the G_0 phase of the cell cycle, cells are in a growth arrest or non-proliferating state. Labile cells continuously proliferate, thus renewing cell populations.
   d. **True.** The renal tubular epithelial cells are good examples of stable cells. This is clinically important. Renal failure caused by tubular damage can resolve, as long as salt–water and acid–base balance can be maintained over this time to allow regeneration of tubular cells and normal renal function to be restored.
   e. **False.** Permanent cells such as neurones and cardiac muscle cells cannot divide. Hyperplasia can, therefore, only occur in labile or stable cell populations.

2. a. **False.** The limiting factor for muscle hypertrophy is the blood supply. A high-protein diet may improve the cellular nutrition to a certain extent, but this cannot continue indefinitely.
   b. **False.** Smoking leads to squamous metaplasia of the bronchial epithelium. Metaplasia is the process where a differentiated epithelium is replaced by another differentiated cell type.
   c. **True.** In pregnancy, there is a massive hormonal stimulus to the breast epithelium which leads to physiological hyperplasia and milk production. When hormone levels return to normal, lactation ceases and the epithelium returns to normal. Hyperplasia is a reversible process. Post-lactation, superfluous cells will be removed by apoptosis.
   d. **True.** Some ovarian cancers can produce large amounts of oestrogen. The endometrium is a target epithelium of oestrogen and under the influence of excess, unopposed oestrogen will undergo hyperplasia. This may persist and become pathological and atypical, and ultimately lead to malignant (cancerous) change.
   e. **False.** Hepatocytes are stable cells. They can regenerate as long as the connective tissue architecture is intact.

3. a. **False.** Atrophy may involve death by apoptosis (individual programmed cell death) but necrosis does not occur.
   b. **False.** Metaplasia is a reversible adaptive response. Removal of the adverse stimulus will result in restitution of the normal tissue. In some cases, a persistent stimulus will lead to neoplastic change. In cigarette smokers, the metaplastic squamous bronchial epithelium becomes increasingly abnormal and eventually squamous cell carcinoma develops.
   c. **True.** Many growth factors are mitogenic — that is they stimulate cells to divide. Examples are epidermal growth factor (EGF), which causes liver and renal epithelial cells to divide, and platelet-derived growth factor (PDGF), which stimulates fibroblasts and smooth muscle cells. However, apparently paradoxically, some growth factors can actually inhibit cell growth; for example, transforming growth factor beta (TGFβ) and tumour necrosis factor (TNF). It is probably the balance between these types of growth factor which contributes to the stability of a cell population.
   d. **False.** Hypertension leads to left ventricular hypertrophy because of increased cardiac muscle fibre size, not an increase in cell numbers. Cardiac muscle cells are permanent cells.
   e. **True.** Interphase is the period between mitoses in the cell cycle. It is the variability in the length of time of G_1 which is mainly responsible for the difference in cell cycle time. The time taken for mitosis (1/2 to 1 hour) is fairly constant in most labile and stable cells.

Case history answers

Case history 1

1. Labile cells. Cytotoxic agents are used in the treatment of some cancers. They act by blocking the cell cycle at various points, preventing cell division. It is not usually possible to target the drugs specifically at the cancer cells, and normal populations of labile cells, such as in the bone marrow, gut epithelium and skin, will also be killed.

2. This example of a child with acute leukaemia shows how a knowledge of the cell cycle and an understanding of cell turnover and proliferation is fundamental to clinical medicine. The effects of cytotoxic drugs are entirely predictable. Normal labile cells, as well as tumour cells, will be destroyed by the cytotoxic drugs. The child will lose his hair (labile hair root cells) and may suffer from gastrointestinal upsets as a result of destruction of gut epithelium. Loss of red cell stem cells leads to anaemia and loss of white cell stem cells predisposes to infection.

3. Cytotoxic drugs are often given in these 'pulses' with drug-free intervals. The rationale behind this is two-fold. Firstly, only a proportion of the rapidly dividing tumour cells will be destroyed by the drugs. During the drug-free time, the tumour cell population re-expands, only to be killed again by the next drug schedule. This maximises the amount of tumour killed. Secondly, a drug-free period between therapies allows some restoration of normal, labile cell numbers, particularly normal bone marrow stem cells.

Case history 2

1. Osteoporosis is an extremely common and important condition in which there is reduction of total bone mass, i.e. bone atrophy, which causes weakening. It is most common in elderly females and predisposes to fractures, especially of the neck of the femur.

   Osteoporosis may be localised to a single bone, e.g. after immobilisation in a plaster cast, or may affect many bones in a generalised way. It is the latter form which is seen in elderly post-menopausal women. In its advanced stages, osteoporosis may be seen on radiographs as pallor or thinning of the bones. The pathogenesis of the disease is not completely understood. However, the main risk factors and associated conditions are:

   - increasing age
   - lack of oestrogen (post-menopausal women)
   - immobilisation after either after fracture or paralysis
   - corticosteroid therapy, where increased bone resorption probably occurs.

2. It is important for this lady to become mobile as quickly as possible post-operatively because she needs to prevent further worsening of the osteoporotic process which might lead to further fractures. She needs to develop muscle tone in her legs to prevent muscle atrophy from immobilisation and also to prevent the development of venous stasis and deep vein thrombosis. In addition, there are important social reasons for her to regain mobility and return home to an independent life.

Short notes answers

1. First of all define both the terms and then highlight what is different and what is similar about them. Use diagrams wherever possible because these are easy to remember and can make your answer more succinct. The subsidiary questions can then be answered simply, referring to the diagrams. Remember, in hyperplasia, once the physiological or pathological stimulus is removed, cell numbers return to normal by apoptosis.

2. Again first define the term 'atrophy', divide it up into 'physiological' and 'pathological' groups and then use a diagram to illustrate the process.

Viva answers

1. **Atrophy** is a reduction in size of an organ as a result of a reduction in size of cells and individual cell death (apoptosis). It is reversible and can have a number of causes, for example, denervation, reduction in hormones or immobilisation. Describe the appearance of atrophic cells, the relationship with apoptosis and the role of lipofuscin.

   Hypertrophy is the increase in size of an organ as a result of an increase in the size of the individual cells. It is reversible and is caused by increased workload, for example in cardiac muscle in hypertension or in skeletal muscle in exercise. Describe the histological appearance of the cells (the cytoplasmic and nuclear components are often perceptibly enlarged down the microscope) and the limiting factors to hypertrophy.

   Hyperplasia is an increase in organ size caused by an increase in the number of constituent cells. It is reversible. Examples are the breast in pregnancy and the stimulated thyroid gland. Discuss physiological versus pathological hyperplasia and the cell types most likely to develop hyperplasia, e.g. labile cells.

2. The cell cycle is the process by which cells synthesise DNA and divide; it can take from as little as 8 hours to several months. Describe the order of events, G_1 through to M and the events that occur at each stage. Mention G_0. Discuss control mechanisms — growth factors and cyclins — and examples of cell populations with different relationships to the cell cycle (i.e. labile, stable and permanent cells). You can also mention the correlation with physiological/pathological hyperplasia and hypertrophy.

3. Regeneration occurs in labile cell populations, which are able to undergo hyperplasia, for example after superficial damage to the gut epithelium or epidermis. It occurs in the absence of structural damage and the outcome is 'good as new'.

   Repair is the result of inflammation and structural damage and involves formation of scar tissue (collagen) from granulation tissue. Permanent cells are usually involved. It is important to remember that even labile and stable cells cannot regenerate if the extracellular matrix of the tissue is damaged.

4. Labile cells proliferate continuously, have a short life span and a high regenerative capacity, for example the cells of bone marrow and gut epithelium.

   Stable cells divide infrequently; they are normally in G_0, the 'non-proliferative' stage of the cell cycle. When stable cells are lost, others in the tissue can regenerate, re-entering the cell cycle at G_1. This re-entry is stimulated by growth factors. Examples of stable cells are hepatocytes and renal epithelial cells.

   Permanent cells divide only in fetal life and cannot be replaced when lost; they are said to be terminally differentiated as they cannot be stimulated to re-enter the cell cycle. Injury to permanent cells cannot be healed by regeneration but only by repair. Examples of permanent cells are neurones and cardiac muscle cells.

Cell injury

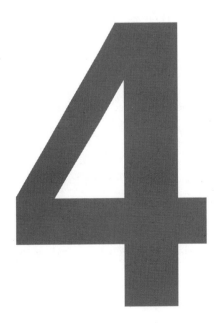

Chapter overview

Cell injury may be reversible (sublethal) or irreversible (lethal). Many causes may result in reversible injury initially, but if severely injured, the cell may be unable to recover and cell death (necrosis or apoptosis) follows.

4.1 Processes involved in cell injury

Causes of cell injury

The causes of both reversible and irreversible cell injury are similar. Many of those listed below may result initially in reversible injury. If the injury is of sufficient severity, e.g. length of exposure to radiation or reduced oxygen supply, the cell reaches a 'point of no return' and irreversible injury culminating in cell death will occur.

Possible causes include:

- hypoxia, e.g. myocardial ischaemia (reduced blood flow to, and therefore oxygenation of, the heart) as a result of coronary artery atherosclerosis
- immunological, e.g. thyroid damage caused by autoantibodies (antibodies produced by the body against its own tissues)
- infection, e.g. bacterial, viral, fungal infections, etc. (e.g. tuberculous infection of the lung)
- genetic, e.g. Duchenne muscular dystrophy
- physical, e.g. sunburn (UV light) damage to the skin
- genetic, e.g. sickle cell disease
- chemical, e.g. acid damage to oesophageal mucosa (accidental or deliberate).

Mechanisms of cell injury

The structure and metabolic function of the cell are interdependent. Therefore, although an injurious agent may target a particular aspect of cell structure or function, this will rapidly lead to wide-ranging secondary effects. Recognised mechanisms of cell injury include:

- cell membrane damage
  - complement-mediated lysis via the membrane attack complex (MAC)
  - bacterial toxins
  - free radicals

- mitochondrial damage leading to inadequate aerobic respiration
  - hypoxia (lack of oxygen)
  - cyanide poisoning

- ribosomal damage leading to altered protein synthesis
  - alcohol in liver cells
  - antibiotics in bacteria

- nuclear damage
  - viruses
  - radiation
  - free radicals.

Free radicals and cell membrane damage

Free radicals are highly reactive atoms which have an unpaired electron in an outer orbital. They can be produced in cells in response to a variety of processes, including radiation, normal metabolic oxidation reactions and drug metabolism processes. The most important free radicals are derived from oxygen, e.g. superoxide and hydroxyl ions. Free radicals can injure cells by generating chain reactions, producing further free radicals, which cause cell membrane damage by cross-linking of proteins and by critical alterations of lipids.

Consequences of cell injury

The consequences of cell injury depend on both the cell and the injurious agent. Certain features of cells make them more vulnerable to serious sequelae of cell injury.

Cell features

Specialisation. Cells that are enzyme rich, nucleated or have specialised organelles within the cytoplasm may be more vulnerable. The presence of specialised proteins within the cell may make it prone to certain types of injurious agent.

Cell state. Cells that have an inadequate supply of oxygen, hormones or growth factors or lack essential nutrients may be more prone to injury.

Regenerative ability. The potential of a cell population to enter the cell cycle and divide is important in the response of tissues to injury. Damaged areas in tissues made up of cells which can divide will quickly be restored to normal, while populations of permanent cells will be incapable of regeneration.

Injury features

In addition, the character of the injury will also affect the severity of the damage.

Type of injury. The injury may be ischaemic, toxic, chemical, etc. Different cells will be more susceptible to some injurious agents than others (e.g. heart muscle cells are more susceptible to oxygen depletion than connective tissue cells).

Exposure time. The length of time of exposure to a toxin or reduced oxygen concentration will affect the chance of a cell surviving the insult, even for those cells relatively resistant to the damaging agent.

Severity. The ability to survive an injury will also depend upon its severity, e.g. is the lack of oxygen partial (hypoxia) or complete (anoxia).

Irreversible cell injury

When does reversible injury become irreversible? The exact 'point of no return' from reversible to irreversible cell injury (leading to cell death) has not yet been defined, although severe mitochondrial damage and cell membrane destruction via free radical generation have been proposed. The light microscopical changes seen in injured cells are well described.

Early changes. These are reversible and include:

- cytoplasmic swelling and vacuolation
- mitochondrial and endoplasmic reticulum swelling
- clumping of nuclear chromatin.

Late changes. These are irreversible and include:

- densities in mitochondrial matrix
- cell membrane disruption
- nuclear shrinkage (pyknosis)
- nuclear dissolution (karyolysis)
- nuclear break up (karyorrhexis)
- lysosome rupture.

4.2 Cell death

Autolysis

Autolysis is the death of individual cells and tissues after the death of the whole organism. The cells are degraded by the post-mortem release of digestive enzymes from the cytoplasmic lysosomes.

Apoptosis

It is now known that cell death encompasses a spectrum of cellular processes. At one end of the spectrum there is **necrosis** where the accidental death of a large number of cells causes an inflammatory response. At the opposite end of the spectrum (some believe) is **apoptosis**. This form of cell death occurs in physiological and embryological processes and appears to be a phenomenon whereby tissues control cell population numbers (sometimes called programmed cell death) or pathological processes (inflammation, cancers) in an attempt by the body to arrest cell proliferation and tissue damage.

During apoptosis, the cell activates genes which code for new proteins, many of which contribute to the cell's own death. The enzyme **endonuclease** is produced or activated, causing DNA fragmentation. In contrast to necrosis, apoptotic cells remain viable and their membrane pumps continue to function until the terminal stages of the process. During apoptosis, the cell shrinks, the nuclear chromatin condenses and the cell breaks into a large number of 'apoptotic bodies'. These can be disposed of by phagocytosis, either by macrophages or, uniquely, by neighbouring normal cells (Fig. 7). Phagocytes recognise apoptotic cells by the new membrane signals which they express. It is important to note that apoptosis does *not* provoke an inflammatory response.

Physiological apoptosis. This can occur in a number of situations:

- embryogenesis: formation of digits
- menstrual cycle: endometrial cell loss
- breast feeding: reversal of changes in the lactating breast once breast feeding is finished
- immune cell development: deletion of immune cells (T cells) that may react with the body's own tissues.

Pathological apoptosis. Individual cell death occurs in a number of pathological conditions:

- tumours (often accompanied by necrosis)
- atrophy (virtually never accompanied by necrosis)
- viral illness (e.g. hepatitis — individual hepatocytes can be seen in apoptotic forms).

The control of apoptosis is crucial in the process of neoplasia. Some genes involved in cancer formation

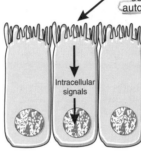

Physiological or pathological insult triggers cell to activate/synthesise autodestructive enzymes

Intracellular signals

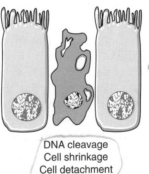

Triggered enzymes may cause changes in cell morphology

DNA cleavage
Cell shrinkage
Cell detachment

Surface signal

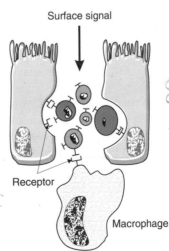

Cell disrupts into 'apoptotic bodies' which may be engulfed by neighbouring normal cells or 'professional' phagocytes i.e. macrophages

Receptor

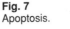
Macrophage

Fig. 7
Apoptosis.

(e.g. the bcl-2 oncogene) seem to be able to switch off apoptosis, allowing cells to live forever.

Necrosis

Necrosis is defined as the morphological changes that result from cell death within living tissues. In necrosis, death of a large number of cells in one area occurs, as opposed to the selective cell death of apoptosis (Fig. 8). These changes occur because of digestion and denaturation of cellular proteins. In fact, the final appearance of the necrotic area will depend on the balance between these two processes. There are several forms of necrosis (see below).

The results of cell death can include:

- cessation of function of a tissue or organ
- release of cellular enzymes; these can sometimes be detected in the blood and used as markers of the extent or timing of damage to a particular organ, e.g. cardiac enzymes after myocardial infarction
- initiation of the inflammatory response (vital reaction).

Types of necrosis

There are five main types of necrosis (Fig. 9):

- coagulative
- caseous
- liquefaction
- fat
- gangrenous.

Coagulative necrosis. Denaturation of intracellular protein (analogous to boiling the white of an egg) leads to the pale firm nature of the tissues affected. The cells show the microscopic features of cell death but the general architecture of the tissue and cell ghosts remain discernible for a short time. Coagulative necrosis is typically seen in the kidney and heart and is usually caused by ischaemia.

Caseous necrosis. This type of cell death is only seen in tuberculosis (TB). The creamy white appearance of the dead tissue is probably a result of the accumulation of partly digested waxy lipid cell wall components of the TB organisms. The tissue architecture is completely destroyed.

Liquefaction necrosis. This results from release of hydrolytic lysosomal enzymes and leads to an accumulation of semi-fluid tissue. It is usually seen in the brain.

Fat necrosis. This can result from direct trauma (common in the fatty tissues of the female breast) or enzyme release from the diseased pancreas. Adipocytes rupture and released fat undergoes lipolysis catalysed by lipases. Macrophages ingest the oily material and a giant cell inflammatory reaction may follow (see Ch. 9). Another consequence is the combination of calcium with the released fatty acids.

Gangrenous necrosis (gangrene). This life-threatening condition occurs when coagulative necrosis of tissues is associated with superadded infection by putrefactive bacteria. These are usually anaerobic Gram-positive *Clostridia* spp. derived from the gut or soil which thrive in conditions of low oxygen tension. Gangrenous tissue is foul smelling and black. The bacteria produce toxins which destroy collagen and enable the infection to spread rapidly. If fermentation occurs, gas gangrene ensues and infection can become systemic (i.e. reach the bloodstream, septicaemia). The commonest clinical situation is gangrene of the lower limb caused by a poor blood supply and superimposed bacterial infection. This is a life-threatening emergency and the limb should be amputated.

A	B
Necrosis **Pro-inflammatory**	**Apoptosis** **Non-inflammatory**

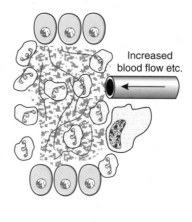

Increased blood flow etc.

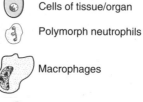

Cells of tissue/organ

Polymorph neutrophils

Macrophages

Apoptotic cell

Fig. 8
Diagrammatic comparison of necrosis and apoptosis.

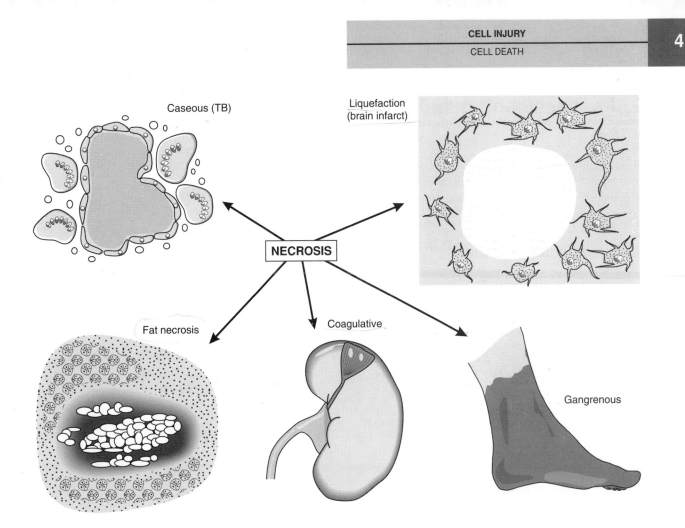

Fig. 9
Types of necrosis.

Self-assessment: quesitons

Topics relating to cell injury are often asked in multiple choice questions or vivas. However, necrosis is a common short notes question — particularly the types of necrosis.

Multiple choice questions

1. The following statements are correct:
   a. Caseous necrosis is characteristically caused by ischaemia
   b. Carbon tetrachloride causes cell injury through free radicals
   c. Disaggregation of polyribosomes is an ultrastructural feature of reversible cell injury
   d. The brain is a common site for gangrenous necrosis
   e. Autolysis is characterised by a vital reaction to dead cells

2. Apoptotic cells:
   a. Exclude vital dyes
   b. Provoke an acute inflammatory reaction
   c. May be disposed of by neighbouring cells
   d. Contain enzymatically degraded nuclear fragments
   e. May be seen in areas of tissue necrosis

3. The following are correctly paired:
   a. Gangrene — anaerobic bacteria
   b. Karyorrhexis — reversible cell injury
   c. Fatty change — alcohol
   d. Free radicals — cell membrane damage
   e. Venous infarction — testicular torsion

Case history

A 59-year-old man, a heavy smoker for much of his adult life, was brought into Casualty at 4 a.m. with a 3-hour history of crushing, band-like chest pain. He was seen immediately but died whilst being examined. His past medical history included diet-controlled (type 2) diabetes mellitus, hypertension and intermittent claudication. He had had several attacks of chest pain over the 5 years before his death. A post-mortem examination was performed.

1. What is the likely cause of death?
2. At post-mortem, the pathologist found no evidence of acute myocardial infarction. Why was this?
3. What changes might have been present in the heart muscle and coronary arteries?
4. How does the medical and social history relate to his terminal event?

Short notes

1. Write short notes on necrosis.

Essay question

1. Discuss the statement 'In ischaemia, influx of calcium into the cell is the point at which injury cannot be reversed'.

Viva questions

1. Define necrosis. How does this differ from autolysis?
2. Describe the main categories of necrosis with examples.
3. Define infarction. Give examples.
4. What are free radicals and how do they cause cell injury?

Self-assessment: answers

Multiple choice answers

1. a. **False.** Caseous necrosis only occurs as a response to TB infection.
   b. **True.** Carbon tetrachloride poisoning is one of the prototypic examples of free radical-induced injury.
   c. **True.** Although electron microscopy is rarely used to examine cell injury/death in day-to-day pathology, it is important to have a working knowledge of the ultrastructural appearances of reversible and irreversible cell injury, if only for exam purposes.
   d. **False.** Gangrenous necrosis characteristically occurs when a tissue/organ that has a resident population of bacteria dies. The organisms then can invade the tissues; depending upon the amount of liquefaction caused by the bacteria, the gangrene is termed 'dry' or 'wet'.
   e. **False.** Autolysis is the process by which post-mortem tissues liquefy as a result of cellular autodigestion. There is no inflammatory reaction to this process (unlike necrosis). Inflammation (see Ch. 9) can *only* occur in *living* and *vascularised* tissues.

2. a. **True.** One of the essential differences between a necrotic and apoptotic cell is that the latter remains 'alive' until late on in the process. Therefore, some dyes, which enter dead cells, are excluded by apoptotic cells.
   b. **False.** Apoptotic cells are disposed of by neighbouring, similar cells or macrophages. No acute inflammation occurs; therefore, tissue damage does not occur.
   c. **True.** See answer (b).
   d. **True.** Soon after apoptosis is triggered, nuclear material in the apoptotic cell is chopped up by endonucleases.
   e. **True.** The processes of necrosis and apoptosis are not mutually exclusive; in particular, apoptotic tumour cells are often seen at the invasion edge of a cancer where extensive necrosis may also be apparent.

3. a. **True.** Gangrenous necrosis is caused by infection of ischaemic necrotic tissues by anaerobic bacteria such as the Gram-positive bacillus *Clostridium welchii*. The bacteria may produce enzymes such as collagenases and hyaluronidases which enables them to spread through tissues planes.
   b. **False.** Karyorrhexis is when the nucleus fragments, denoting severe irreversible cell injury.

   c. **True.** Fatty change is commonly seen in liver cells which have been damaged by alcohol. The cells accumulate triglycerides as droplets within the cell cytoplasm, rather than exporting them complexed to proteins in the form of lipoproteins. Fatty change is reversible.
   d. **True.** Free radicals seem to be one of the final common pathways of cell damage and affect the cell membrane and the nuclear DNA.
   e. **True.** Torsion (twisting) of the testis on its cord leads to a reduction in the arterial flow to the organ combined with obstruction to the venous drainage. The infarct is haemorrhagic and fills the testis with venous blood. Infarction of the testis can be prevented if the cord can be untwisted as soon as possible. This is not an uncommon surgical emergency in young men with sudden pain in the testis. Venous infarction can also be seen in the ovary and the gut.

Case history answer

1. The likely cause of death in this man is ischaemic heart disease caused by coronary artery atherosclerosis. The chest pain he describes is quite characteristic of pain owing to an ischaemic myocardium (heart muscle deprived of blood supply and thus oxygen). Severe atherosclerosis (furring up) of his coronary arteries would account for this.

2. This is an important point. The macroscopic (naked eye) and microscopic changes that characterise all forms of necrosis take time to develop (see p. 32). There is a significant lag, in this and in any case, between the onset of ischaemia and any changes in the myocardium that can be seen by the naked eye. This is not an unusual scenario at autopsy. A patient who has died instantly from myocardial ischaemia (clinically causing a lethal abnormal heart rhythm such as ventricular fibrillation) because of complete blockage of one or more coronary artery will have no evidence of acute infarction. If, however, the patient had lived for 3–4 days after this event and then died, established myocardial necrosis with its attendant inflammatory response would be seen: a pale and haemorrhagic area with typical microscopic features of cell death and inflammation.

3. The history of previous attacks of chest pain suggest past ischaemic events and the pathologist may find fibrosis (scarring) of the myocardium because cardiac muscle cells are permanent cells and regeneration cannot occur. The man suffered from hypertension (high blood pressure); therefore, hypertrophy of the myocardium is likely. The normal heart weighs about 250–350 g, but in severe

hypertension the weight can double and much of this will be because of hypertrophy of the left ventricular myocardium. The coronary arteries will be atherosclerotic (see answers 2 and 4).

4. The pathological process that led to this man's death was atherosclerosis and he had several important risk factors for this, namely smoking, hypertension and type 2 diabetes mellitus. The fact that he suffered from intermittent claudication (cramping pains in the calves, usually caused by exertion-induced muscle ischaemia and, therefore, oxygen lack because of atherosclerotic limb arteries) emphasises the widespread nature of this process.

Short notes answer

1. Irrespective of the length or detail of the written answer, always begin by defining the term, in this case 'necrosis'. Then outline the classification with examples of the causes, appearances (naked eye and down the microscope) and long-term consequences or complications of the processes.

Essay answer

1. This type of question should only be tackled if you have a good working knowledge of the cellular events in reversible and irreversible cell injury (Fig. 10). Damage to the mitochondria is only one of several theories as to the 'final straw' that breaks the cell's ability to reverse the injury it has suffered.

Viva answers

1. Necrosis is the death of cells within the living body:

   - causes: ischaemia, trauma, infection, immunological injury, chemicals
   - types: coagulative, gangrenous, fat, liquefactive, caseous
   - consequences: enzyme release, e.g. creatine kinase (CK) after myocardial infarction — total CK levels in the blood will start to rise about 5 hours after a heart attack and peak at about 36 hours
   - inflammatory reaction follows: healing and repair.

   Autolysis is the death of cells and tissues after the death of the whole organism. Autolysis results from the release of lytic enzymes from lysosomes.

2. There are five types of necrosis:

   - coagulative: denaturation of intracellular protein, typically seen in the kidney and heart and is usually caused by ischaemia; it is important to note that there is preservation of cell outlines
   - caseous: tissue architecture destroyed with a characteristic vital reaction around it, only seen in

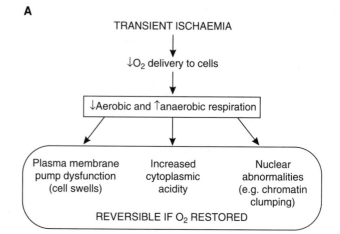

A

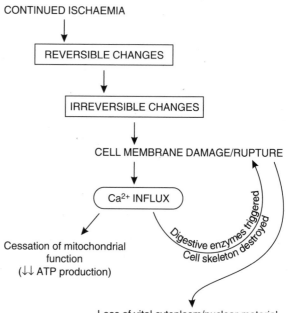

Fig. 10
Cellular events in reversible and irreversible injury.

tuberculosis; in caseous necrosis, cell outlines are not apparent

- liquefactive: accumulation of semi-fluid tissue through the action of lysosomal enzymes, usually seen in the brain
- fat: adipocytes rupture releasing fats that are broken down—the oily material can be ingested by macrophages to give a foreign body giant cell reaction or combine with calcium; fat necrosis can result from direct trauma, e.g. in the breast, or from pancreatic diseases, e.g. acute pancreatitis
- gangrenous: infection of coagulative necrotic tissue by putrefactive anaerobic bacteria (*Clostridia* spp.); toxins destroy collagen and fermentation produces gases leading to systemic infection; it occurs most often in the lower limb; if there is marked liquefaction of the tissues (as a

result of the bacteria or inflammatory reaction) the appearance is often referred to as 'wet gangrene'.

3. Infarction is the death of tissue within the living body, due to ischaemia (lack of oxygen supply). Myocandial infarction is the death of cardiac muscle as a result of occlusion of coronary arteries by atherosclerosis and/or thrombosis.

4. Free radicals are highly reactive atoms which have an unpaired election. They can injure cells by generating a chain reaction of free radical productions which causes cell membrane damage by cross linking of proteins and alterations to membrane lipids.

Cascades, haemostasis and shock

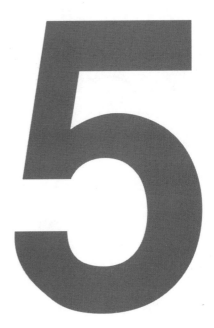

Chapter overview

Cascade systems occur frequently in the body, particularly in the immune and haemostatic processes. Malfunction in any part of a cascade can lead to disease. Shock is an ill-defined series of changes which occur after severe and sudden diminution in the blood volume or cardiac output. The common feature of all causes of shock is substantially reduced circulating volume.

5.1 Principles of cascade systems

Many vascular and cellular processes are triggered by chemical mediators, which are described in various sections of this book. They can be seen in immune, inflammatory and vascular events but they are all inter-related and share the common underlying mechanism of cascade action in which the product of one reaction catalyses the subsequent reaction, thus amplifying the response (Fig. 11). Chemical mediators are present in plasma and in the tissues. Examples of these cascade systems are given in Table 4.

The main characteristics of a cascade system are:

- activation by a tissue event
- a series of enzymatic steps
- inactive precursors are converted to active forms
- powerful action in small concentrations
- each step amplifies the reaction
- rapid breakdown and inactivation of constituents.

The cascades involved in the haemostatic (clotting) complement and fibrinolytic systems are interlinked. Plasmin, a product of the fibrin olytic cascade, degrades the product of the clotting cascade and activates complement. Hageman factor, or factor XII, is a clotting fac-

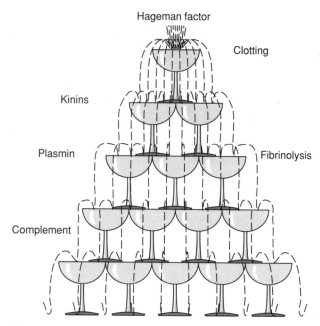

Fig. 11
Cascades: illustrating the principles of activation and amplification.

tor which activates the complement, kinase and fibrinolytic systems (Fig. 11).

5.2 The complement cascade

The complement cascade forms an important part of the body's defence system against microbial infection (Fig. 12). It interacts with the antibody response and with the inflammatory process. Complement reactions are triggered by:

- antigen–antibody complexes (classical pathway)
- Gram-negative bacterial endotoxin, i.e. surface complex molecules (alternative pathway).

Table 4 Cascade systems

	Activator	End product	Function
Kinin system	Hageman factor (factor XII)	Bradykinin	Vasodilatation/hypotension, increased vascular permeability
Complement system	Antigen–antibody complexes	C3a/C5a	Chemotaxis, increased vascular permeability
		Membrane attack complex (C5b–9)	Cell lysis
	Endotoxin (bacterial surfaces)	C3b	Opsonisation
Clotting system	Endothelial damage	Fibrin	Haemostasis (platelet–fibrin plug)
	Hageman factor	Fibrinopeptides	Increased vascular permeability
Fibrinolytic system	Plasminogen activator from endothelium	Plasmin	Lysis of fibrin clots Degrades fibrin to form fibrin degradation products (FDPs)

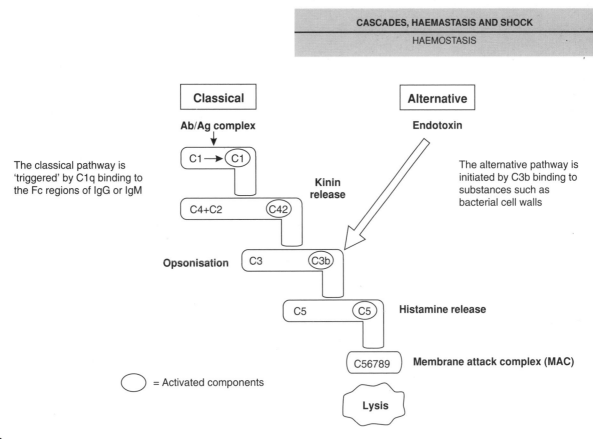

Fig. 12
Complement cascade. Ab/Ag, antibody–antigen complex; complement components have C numbers, e.g. C1.

Complement assists in defence in three ways

- **triggering acute inflammation**: C3a, C5a — the anaphylatoxins — cause histamine-mediated vasodilatation and blood vessel leakage as well as acting as potent chemotaxins for neutrophils and monocytes
- **helping phagocytosis** by coating foreign substances, e.g. bacterial cell walls, with protein (opsonisation)
- **direct killing** of certain organisms: MAC formation may kill some bacteria, e.g. *Neisseria* spp.

Complement activation can lead to extensive tissue damage and plays an important part in hypersensitivity reactions (Ch. 8).

The **classical** pathway of complement activation occurs when antigen and antibody (IgG or IgM) combine to form a complex. The **alternative** pathway activates complement without IgG or IgM being present, i.e. bacterial lipopolysaccharides (endotoxin), snake venom or aggregated IgA are the triggers.

5.3 Haemostasis

Blood clotting

The blood vessel wall, platelets and the clotting cascade are the three major components of normal blood clotting (haemostasis).

Blood vessel wall
Normal continuous endothelium inhibits intravascular clotting by preventing blood platelets from coming into contact with the collagen of the vessel wall. Endothelial cells also produce substances such as prostaglandins (PGI_2), nitric oxide and plasminogen activator which inhibit platelet aggregation and promote fibrinolysis. If the endothelium is damaged and collagen is exposed to the blood, then thrombogenic tissue factors will trigger the clotting cascade, leading to fibrin clot formation.

Platelets
Platelets have a central role in clotting and form the initial plug to an area of endothelial damage. To do this they have to adhere to the site of injury (exposed collagen) and then release stored products from granules rich in ADP, platelet-derived growth factor (PDGF), serotonin, calcium and fibrinogen, which trigger platelet aggregation and the clotting cascade. Thromboxane A_2 (TXA_2), synthesised and released by activated platelets, plays a key role in platelet aggregation (Fig. 13). The platelet plug is not a robust structure and thrombin and fibrin are required to stabilise it.

The clotting cascade
The clotting cascade is triggered by:

- exposure of blood to glass or collagen (intrinsic pathway)
- exposure to factors derived from injured cells (extrinsic pathway).

In either case, the pathway leads to thrombin formation. Thrombin converts soluble fibrinogen to insoluble fibrin,

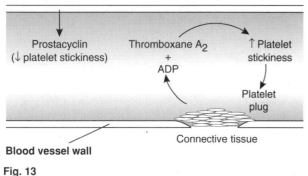

Blood vessel wall

Fig. 13
The platelet plug.

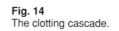

the protein which ultimately stabilises the clot. The overall process is summarised in Figure 14.

Fibrinolysis

The fibrinolytic system is activated alongside the clotting system and results in the production of plasmin, which degrades fibrin and fibrin clots. One of the 'triggers' involved in the activation of the fibrinolytic system is factor XII.

Disseminated intravascular coagulation (DIC)

This is an important condition where both clotting and haemorrhage occur together. The patient is usually very ill because of underlying diseases, such as:

- severe overwhelming infection (septicaemia)
- severe tissue trauma (burns)
- post-partum haemorrhage (massive bleeding after birth).

In all these conditions, there is activation of the coagulation system, by either the extrinsic or intrinsic pathways. Thus, endothelial cells may be damaged in burns and by immune complexes. Tissue factors may be released by the placenta. This mass activation of the clotting cascade leads to the consumption of vast amounts of platelets and fibrin. The formation of multiple platelet thrombi occurs in the microvasculature. These cause small areas of infarction in many organs.

At the same time the fibrinolytic system is activated and thrombi are rapidly dissolved, producing large amounts of fibrin degradation products. Supplies of clotting factors and platelets may become exhausted (consumption coagulopathy) so that a paradoxical situation occurs, where there is disseminated thrombosis with multi-organ infarcts and haemorrhage. DIC is a serious life-threatening illness which needs to be managed by treating the underlying cause (e.g. antibiotics for infection) and by replacement of clotting factors and anticoagulants.

Collagen/test tube   Tissue injury/tissue factor production

Fig. 14
The clotting cascade.

5.4 Shock

Shock is a series of changes which occur after a severe and sudden reduction in circulating blood volume, often a consequence of diminished cardiac output, commonly as a result of acute major damage. The body attempts to maintain an adequate blood supply to essential organs such as the brain. The end result is low perfusion hypoxic injury to cells and tissues. For example, the kidneys may undergo acute tubular necrosis, the heart may develop subendocardial necrosis and the gut may become ischaemic.

The most usual syndrome of shock consists of:

- hypotension (low blood pressure)
- weak thready pulse
- tachycardia (fast heart rate)
- clammy cold skin.

Shock can be subdivided into various types depending upon the initiating 'injury'.

Hypovolaemic shock. This occurs after severe haemorrhage, e.g. traumatic damage or severing of a major artery, or loss of body fluids such as water from the colon in cholera or from the skin in burns cases. Major vasoconstriction occurs to preserve blood flow to the heart and brain.

Cardiogenic shock. This usually occurs secondary to myocardial infarction, rupture of a cardiac valve cusp or arrhythmia, but it can also occur through any cause of 'pump' failure.

Septic (endotoxic) shock. Circulatory failure occurs as the result of major bacterial infection, usually with Gram-negative bacteria such as *Escherichia coli*, *Klebsiella* or *Pseudomonas* spp. In contrast to hypovolaemic and cardiogenic shock, patients may be vasodilated (and feel warm). Vascular damage occurs through the action of endotoxins, produced by the bacteria, and of kinins.

Anaphylactic shock. This occurs as a result of an acute systemic type 1 hypersensitivity reaction in people who are sensitised to the antigen, e.g. penicillin. It is a severe rapid reaction with bronchospasm, laryngeal oedema and hypotension.

Neurogenic shock. This may be caused by damage to the spinal cord, with peripheral vasodilatation and pooling of blood.

Self-assessment: questions

Multiple choice questions

1. The following statements are true:
   a. C5a of the complement system causes opsonisation
   b. Plasmin can activate complement via the classical pathway
   c. Clotting factor XII is also known as the Hageman factor
   d. Factor VIII deficiency (haemophilia) leads to defective haemostasis
   e. Plasma fibrinogen is insoluble

2. The following statements are correct:
   a. Fibrin is a soluble protein
   b. Clotting factor VIII requires vitamin K for its synthesis
   c. The intrinsic coagulation pathway is triggered by exposed collagen
   d. Platelet aggregation is promoted by thromboxane A_2
   e. Disseminated intravascular coagulation (DIC) results in an increase in the amounts of measurable clotting factors in the plasma

Case history

A 59-year-old male lorry driver was involved in a road traffic accident in which he sustained severe injuries to the head and pelvis. On admission to hospital, he was unconscious and hypotensive (BP 60/30 mmHg). He was cold and clammy and had a pulse rate of 150 per minute. He was transfused with eight units of blood. He underwent extensive surgery for a fractured pelvis and ruptured pelvic blood vessels and his condition stabilised. Over the next few days, he regained consciousness, but it was noticed that he was not passing urine. Blood tests showed that he was in renal failure. He then developed a fever and infection of his pelvic wounds. Gram-negative bacteria were cultured from his blood and again he became hypotensive, tachycardic and peripherally cyanosed. Despite antibiotic treatment he died.

1. What is the likely cause of shock in this patient?
2. Why did he develop renal failure?
3. What are the mechanisms involved in the development of septicaemic shock?
4. If he had survived, what would have happened to his renal function?

Short notes

Write short notes on the following:

1. The main factors required for normal haemostasis
2. The process of opsonisation and phagocytosis; why are these processes important?

Self-assessment: answers

Multiple choice answers

1. a. **False.** Opsonisation is the process whereby foreign material, e.g. microorganisms, become coated with natural protein before ingestion by neutrophils or macrophages. The two main opsonins are C3b and the Fc fragment of IgG. This function of C3b is of great biological value to the host because invading organisms can be opsonised even if it is the first exposure to that infection. The C3b-coated organism is recognised by receptors on the cell surface.
   b. **True.** This is an important link between the clotting and complement systems. Hageman factor (clotting factor XII) can activate the complement, kinin and fibrinolytic systems.
   c. **True.** This is the important linking factor between all the cascade systems.
   d. **True.** Haemophilia is an X-linked genetic disorder, which means that it is mainly clinically apparent in males. It is caused by a lack of factor VIII, which means that the clotting cascade is inefficient and effective haemostasis cannot occur. Patients with haemophilia suffer from haemorrhages into joints and tissues, often triggered by relatively minor trauma. They are treated by replacement with fresh frozen plasma or recombinant factor VIII.
   e. **False.** Fibrinogen is the soluble plasma protein which is converted to insoluble thrombus-forming fibrin within the clotting cascade.

2. a. **False.** Fibrinogen is the soluble plasma protein which is the precursor of fibrin. Fibrin is an insoluble fibrillary protein produced by the clotting cascade during haemostasis. It binds the blood clot and seals blood vessel defects.
   b. **False.** Most of the clotting factors are synthesised in the liver, but only factors II, VII, IX and X are vitamin K dependent. Patients with liver disease commonly run into problems with their haemostasis when the diseased liver cannot produce adequate amounts of clotting factors.
   c. **True.** The intrinsic pathway is activated by exposed collagen, i.e. from vessel wall damage or atherosclerosis. It starts with factor XII (Hageman factor) and the cascade progresses quickly through to the formation of thrombin and fibrin.
   d. **True.** Thromboxane A$_2$ is a prostaglandin-like metabolite of arachidonic acid. It enhances platelet aggregation, which is an important step in the process of haemostasis. Arachidonic acid is found in fish oils and ingestion of these is thought to have beneficial effects in preventing thrombosis formation in relation to atherosclerotic plaques.

   e. **False.** In DIC, there is a consumption of clotting factors and platelets, which rapidly become depleted and exacerbate the haemorrhagic complications of this life-threatening disorder.

Case history answer

1. This patient is probably suffering from hypovolaemic shock as a result of massive blood loss from his fractured pelvic bones and torn blood vessels. This type of shock can also be seen in cases of severe gastrointestinal bleeding, such as from bleeding peptic ulcers or oesophageal varices, which are a consequence of alcoholic cirrhosis.
2. He developed renal failure as a consequence of acute tubular necrosis. In severe shock with hypotension, the renal tubules become ischaemic, die and cease to function, leading to acute renal failure. The glomeruli are less susceptible to ischaemia and, therefore, would not be affected.
3. Patients with Gram-negative septicaemia can develop endotoxic shock. Endotoxin (bacterial wall lipopolysaccharides) can directly trigger the alternative complement pathway and this leads to massive release of coagulation factors, pyrogens and kinins as well as stimulation of monocytes and macrophages. These cells will also produce numerous pro-inflammatory molecules, e.g. cytokines and growth factors.

   A distinction should be made between septicaemia, which is a life-threatening condition whereby pathogenic organisms multiply and circulate in the bloodstream, and a bacteraemia, where non-proliferating bacteria circulate in the blood but are easily removed by the body's phagocytic cells. Bacteraemia can occur whenever there is potential for bacteria to enter the blood stream, e.g. after a visit to the dentist, or after any invasive surgical procedure.
4. Renal tubules are lined by epithelial cells, which are stable cells. Therefore, when they become ischaemic and die, they will regenerate as long as the basement membrane and matrix components of the kidney tubules are intact. In clinical practice, as long as the condition is recognised and the patient can be supported with control of fluid, salt and acid–base balance, full recovery will occur. In this patient, however, the superadded septicaemia was the cause of death.

Short notes answers

1. Normal blood clotting and haemostasis require a normal endothelium and normal levels and activities of clotting factors and enzymes. Normal

numbers of functioning platelets are also required. Examples of where things can go wrong include:

Vitamin K deficiency. The clotting factors II, VII, IX and X are vitamin K dependent and their active forms are produced by the liver. Therefore, patients with liver disease may develop a bleeding tendency. Vitamin K deficiency may occur in newborn babies, leading to intracranial haemorrhage.

Thrombocytopenia. Patients who have low levels of circulating platelets will bleed and bruise easily. Autoimmune destruction of platelets or invasion of bone marrow by tumour or treatment with cytotoxic drugs can cause these problems.

Poorly controlled anticoagulant therapy. Inappropriate dosages of anticoagulants can lead to haemorrhage. Heparin is usually given intra-venously for immediate effect whereas warfarin is given orally and takes longer to work. Patients on anticoagulant therapy require regular blood tests to monitor their clotting status.

2. Opsonisation (from Greek meaning to prepare for the table) is the process whereby foreign material is coated with complement or IgG to promote engulfment by phagocytic cells such as macrophages. It is an important part of the immune reaction against bacteria. Bacterial lipopolysaccharides activate complement via the alternative pathway, generating C3b. Antibody binding to bacterial antigens also activates the complement cascade via the classical pathway and additional C3b is produced. Opsonisation helps phagocytosis by promoting adhesion of the bacterial particle to the phagocyte cell surface.

Atherosclerosis and thrombosis

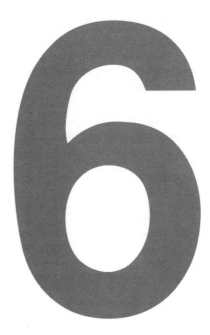

Chapter overview

Atherosclerosis, a common degenerative disease of arteries, characterised by thickening of the intima as a result of deposition of lipids, is the main pathological process that leads to cardiovascular disease.

6.1 Atherosclerosis

Cardiovascular disease gives rise to heart attacks, strokes and aneurysms, which are the major causes of death in the Western world. Atherosclerosis is the pathological process underlying these diseases. It is an acquired, degenerative disease which affects large and medium-sized arteries (e.g. aorta, carotid and coronary arteries), where it begins in the innermost intimal layer. It is characterised by lipid deposition and fibrosis ('scarring'). Atheroma (Grk porridge) is a term which is often used synonymously with atherosclerosis.

The important risk factors for developing atherosclerosis are:

- increasing age
- cigarette smoking
- hypertension
- male sex
- hyperlipidaemia
- diabetes mellitus.

Pathogenesis

The earliest visible lesion of atherosclerosis is the fatty streak which results from accumulation of lipid-laden macrophages within the intima and which can be seen in the arteries of children. Fatty streaks are flat, yellow spots. It is not known with certainty whether these are precursor lesions or atheromatous plaques. Fibrolipid (atheromatous plaques occur later in life and contain macrophages intermingled with proliferating smooth muscle cells, capped by fibrous tissue. Lipid, particularly cholesterol, may be present within both macrophages and smooth muscle cells. Tiny blood vessels can sometimes be seen entering the periphery of the lesions. These plaques actually protrude into the vessel lumen and cause narrowing. Several different theories have been proposed to explain the initiation and evolution of atherosclerosis. The current, favoured idea is the 'response to injury hypothesis', which brings some of these together.

The response to injury hypothesis

Damage to the arterial endothelium leads to increased permeability of the vessel wall and attachment of platelets and monocytes. These produce substances (growth factors) which stimulate smooth muscle cells of the arterial media to migrate into the intima and proliferate. One of these growth factors is platelet-derived growth factor (PDGF). This is a locally acting polypeptide which binds to cell surface receptors and triggers a chain of events which may enable genes to switch on and produce proteins which promote cell proliferation. Proliferating smooth muscle cells produce collagens and proteoglycans, which form the fibrotic cap and matrix of the atherosclerotic plaque. The monocytes transform into macrophages (with or without intracellular lipid — the lipid has entered the leaky vessel wall) within the intima and also produce secretory products, including more growth factors which attract inflammatory cells into and around the plaque (Fig. 15).

Lipids and atherosclerosis

Low density lipoproteins (LDLs) are rich in cholesterol and raised blood levels of LDLs are probably the most important factor in plaque genesis. Both genetic and environmental dietary factors can determine the LDL levels, but the precise mechanism of this relationship with plaque development is not known. Genetic abnormalities can lead to increased blood levels in very young people, who may suffer heart attacks and strokes in their late teens or early 20s. There is a strong epidemiological correlation between cardiovascular disease and high LDL blood levels. In contrast there is a reduced risk of atherosclerosis with high levels of high density lipoproteins (HDLs) containing cholesterol.

Fish oils. Populations which have a high dietary intake of fish oil containing special fatty acids seem to be protected from developing complicated atherosclerosis. Fish oils may have a blood lipid-lowering effect, resulting in reduced levels of LDLs and raised levels of HDLs. Fish oils may also reduce levels of thromboxane A_2, which is metabolised from arachidonic acid in platelets and increases their capacity to aggregate. Reducing thromboxane A_2 levels may reduce the risk of thrombosis.

Complications of atherosclerosis

In many instances, it is not the atherosclerotic plaque itself that is lethal, but that a number of possible events (complications) such as haemorrhage or thrombosis

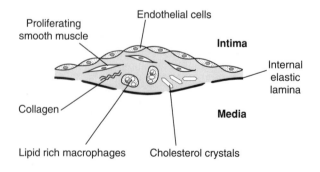

Fig. 15
The fibrolipid plaque in atherosclerosis.

'Uncomplicated' atherosclerosis

Complicated atherosclerosis

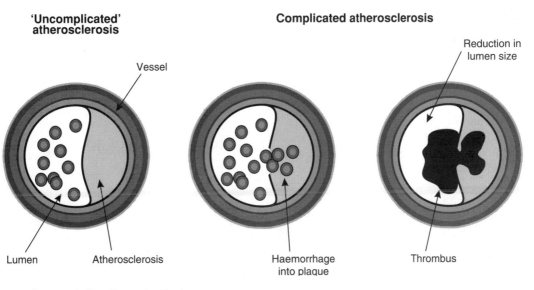

Fig. 16
Complications occurring on or in the atherosclerotic plaque.

may occur in or on the plaque (Fig. 16). Since the plaque is intimal and protrudes into the lumen of the vessel, some of these complications will be serious, causing occlusion (blockage) of the artery and, therefore, death of the tissue supplied. Complications include:

- ulceration and thrombosis
- haemorrhage
- calcification
- aneurysm.

Ulceration and thrombosis
The atherosclerotic plaque usually bulges into the lumen of the artery. Fast-flowing blood may ulcerate the plaque, allowing discharge of its contents or thrombosis to be triggered. The thrombus may occlude the already narrowed lumen. In a vessel such as a coronary or carotid artery, this may prove lethal; occurring in the coronary artery it could cause myocardial infarction and in the cerebral arteries it could cause a stroke.

Haemorrhage
Blood can be forced into the plaque from the lumen of the vessel or bleeding can occur from the vessels vascularising the base and edges of the plaque.

Calcification
Old atherosclerotic plaques often undergo dystrophic calcification. Hence atherosclerotic arteries can some-

times be seen on radiographs (e.g. of the abdomen — abdominal aorta).

Aneurysm formation
The presence of a large, expanding intimal plaque inevitably leads to atrophy and weakening of the arterial media. The weakened vessel wall will dilate and eventually a large sac is formed. This is called an aneurysm. A variety of complications can follow, including rupture, thrombosis and embolism (Fig. 16).

6.2 Thrombosis

This is the process whereby a thrombus is formed. A thrombus is a solid mass composed of blood constituents which develops in an artery or a vein. Thrombus formation can only occur during life. This is in contrast to clotting (haemostasis), which can occur after death or in a test tube. There are three main predisposing factors for thrombus formation (Virchow's triad):

- damage to the endothelial lining of a blood vessel
- relative stasis or turbulence of blood flow
- increased coagulability of blood.

These predisposing factors are associated with particular conditions or life styles (see Table 5).

Table 5 Predisposing factors for thrombosis

	Examples
Endothelial damage	Trauma, atherosclerosis, smoking, bacterial toxins
Stasis/turbulence	Post-operative immobility (inactive legs) and blood pooling; post-myocardial infarction (sluggish blood flow around body); turbulence around atherosclerotic plaques, within aneurysms
Increased coagulability	Pregnancy; oral contraceptives; leukaemia; cancer

How does a thrombus form?

Any of the above factors alone or in combination may predispose to the formation of a thrombus. Thrombi build up from the platelet plug. The clotting cascade is triggered by endothelial damage and factors released by the aggregation of platelets. As the blood flows past, red cells become trapped in the fibrin mesh which is thus formed. The thrombus grows in layers in the direction of the blood flow, a process known as propagation. To the naked eye, a thrombus is a dark red mass of blood in which delicate white lines of fibrin can be seen. These 'lines of Zahn' help to distinguish between a thrombus and a clot. Other distinguishing features are the granularity and relative rigidity of the thrombus and the fact that it may be attached to the vessel wall.

Thrombi can occur in arteries, veins or within the heart chambers (mural thrombus). The outcome of thrombus formation can be:

- propagation leading to complete occlusion of vessel lumen
- removal by fibrinolysis
- organisation and recanalisation (granulation tissue ingrowth, forming capillary channels that traverse the thrombus, allowing blood to flow through it again)
- embolism (breaking off of the thrombus into the circulation to lodge in a distant vessel).

6.3 Embolism

An embolus is a mass of material which is carried in the bloodstream and can become lodged within a blood vessel and block it. The material may be a solid, liquid or a gas. The effects of an embolus follow from the obstruction of blood flow to the tissues and depend on the precise site at which this occurs and whether or not there is an alternative tissue blood supply. Emboli travel through the circulatory system and obstruct the vessel lumen when the diameter prevents further passage. The most common types and sources of embolism are given in Table 6.

Pulmonary embolism

This most commonly arises from a thrombus in the deep leg or pelvic veins. Small emboli may go unnoticed and dissolve by fibrinolysis, whereas a large embolus which lodges in a main pulmonary artery may cause sudden death. Other emboli may cause severe respiratory and cardiac symptoms, relating to either infarction of the lung or right-sided heart strain.

Risk factors for deep vein thrombosis include:

- old age
- immobility
- post-operative state
- late pregnancy and post-partum state
- oral contraceptives
- polycythaemia (increased red cell numbers).

Systemic embolism

Systemic emboli arise in the left side of the heart or in the arterial system and cause death of tissue beyond the occlusion. For example, multiple small embolic showers of atherosclerotic debris from the carotid arteries may lead to temporary loss of blood flow to parts of the brain (transient ischaemic attack). A large piece of mural thrombus detaching from a myocardial infarction could lead to gut, splenic or renal ischaemia by blocking the appropriate artery.

Table 6 Types of embolism and their sources

Type	Source
Thrombus (thrombo-embolus)	Deep vein of leg/pelvis, causes pulmonary embolism Endocardium over a myocardial infarct A fibrillating atrium, when it can lead to systemic embolism
Atherosclerotic plaque debris	Any affected large or medium-size artery: it will embolise to distant sites further 'downstream'
Infective vegetations	Heart valves: right heart valves to lungs, left heart valves to brain or systemic circulation
Amniotic fluid	Uterus at delivery: it can embolise to lungs via torn uterine veins or placenta
Nitrogen	Inadequate decompression in deep-sea divers: emboli cause problems in lungs, heart, spinal cord and skeleton
Air	Deliberate or accidental surgical introduction of air into circulation, e.g. into great veins in chest
Fat	Complicated bony fractures: emboli to lungs, brain and kidney

6.4 Infarction

Infarction is defined as death of tissue caused by ischemia, or lack of oxygen. It may result from a partial or complete reduction of the blood supply (arterial infarction) or diminished drainage of blood from the tissue (venous infarction). The shape and size of the infarct depends on the territory normally supplied or drained by the occluded blood vessel. The appearance of an infarct varies, depending on how long the process has been going on. The vast majority of infarcts are arterial in nature and are caused by thrombosis or embolism.

Direct occlusion of arterial supply (white infarct) occurs as a result of:

- thrombus: coronary artery thrombosis leads to myocardial infarction
- embolus: pulmonary embolus and infarction caused by deep vein thrombosis of the calf
- clamping of an artery during surgery.

Obstruction of venous outflow (red infarct) occurs as a result of:

- twisting or constriction of tissue or organ (e.g. torsion of testis or entrapment of loop of bowel in a hernia sac)
- compression of the vein by a tumour mass.

The appearance of a myocardial infarction changes with time. The macroscopic (visible to the naked eye) and microscopic changes of the resulting necrosis take time to develop (Table 7).

Table 7 Appearances of myocardial infarction

Time after infarct	Naked eye	Microscopic
Less than 24 hours	No visible changes	Cytoplasm looks pinker than normal (eosinophilic)
48 hours	Indistinct pallor or haemorrhage	Necrotic area with acute inflammatory cells at edges
5 days to 2 weeks	Definite pallor, bright red rim	Amorphous, acellular area with macrophages, maturing granulation tissue
3 weeks to months	Pale scar	Mature fibrous scar tissue

Self-assessment: questions

Multiple choice questions

1. The following statements are true:
   a. Mural thrombus in the left ventricle may embolise to the brain
   b. Thrombosis occurs in veins and arteries
   c. Vascular endothelium produces prothrombin
   d. Atherosclerosis only occurs in large arteries with turbulent blood flow
   e. The pale areas in a thrombus are caused by trapped white blood cells

2. The following statements are correct:
   a. Increased levels of high density lipoproteins (HDLs) predispose to atherosclerosis
   b. Dietary cholesterol levels are directly related to plasma cholesterol levels
   c. Atherosclerotic plaques contain proliferating smooth muscle cells
   d. Atherosclerosis is an important cause of aneurysm formation
   e. Thrombus commonly develops on atherosclerotic plaques

3. The following are correctly paired:
   a. Lines of Zahn in a thrombus — white blood cells
   b. Embolus — fragments of thrombus
   c. Abdominal aortic aneurysm — leg ischaemia
   d. Myocardial infarction — ventricular mural thrombus
   e. Cerebral infarction — deep vein thrombosis

Case histories

Case history 1

A 35-year-old woman gave birth to healthy twin babies. She went home after 7 days but was readmitted to hospital 5 days later complaining of feeling breathless with pleuritic chest pain (a sharp stabbing pain in the side of her chest which was worse on breathing in). Her left leg was slightly swollen and she was tender over the calf. Investigations showed that she had a small infarct in the left lower lung lobe. She was treated with the anticoagulant heparin and made a good recovery. She was discharged home on a course of warfarin.

1. What has caused the infarct in her lung (i.e. what is the diagnosis)?
2. What are the risk factors for this condition?
3. Describe the rationale for treatment with heparin and warfarin.

Case history 2

A 68-year-old man was a heavy smoker and presented to his doctor with a painful, black big toe. This was gangrenous on examination and he was admitted to hospital urgently for treatment and surgical amputation. He made a good recovery and was well for a year. He then started to develop pain in the lower back which came and went but was not severe enough to bother his doctor with. On one occasion, however, he experienced excruciating pain in the lower right back and rapidly became shocked and collapsed with a pulse rate of 120/min and a systolic blood pressure of 60 mmHg. He was rushed to hospital but died in the ambulance.

A post-mortem was performed at which a large abdominal aneurysm was found which had ruptured. There were 3 litres of fresh blood clot in the retroperitoneum, tracking up behind the right kidney. The aorta showed severe atherosclerosis elsewhere.

1. How might you connect the episode of gangrene in the toe with the final pathology in this man?
2. What are the main risk factors for atherosclerosis?
3. What are the complications of an abdominal aortic aneurysm?

Short notes

Write short notes on the following:

1. Embolus
2. Risk factors for coronary atherosclerosis
3. Infarction.

Viva questions

1. Discuss thrombosis versus clotting.
2. Discuss modifiable risk factors for atherosclerosis.

Self-assessment: answers

Multiple choice answers

1. a. **True.** Mural thrombus in the left ventricle may develop after myocardial infarction. The dead cardiac muscle and disruption of the endocardium cause thrombosis to occur. If pieces break off and embolise then they can end up anywhere in the systemic circulation. The brain is a common site for this and an embolus travelling through the carotid arteries and then into a cerebral artery will cause ischaemic infarction of the brain (stroke). Cardiac mural thrombus can also embolise and cause infarcts in the spleen, gut or kidney.

   b. **True.** Thrombosis will occur in any vessel in which one or more of the three factors of Virchow's triad have occurred: endothelial damage, increased blood coagulability and altered flow.

   c. **False.** Prothrombin is produced by the liver and is the inactive precursor of thrombin, the protein which causes fibrin to be formed and hence coagulation to occur. Vascular endothelium does produce plasminogen, which tends to counteract any tendency to coagulate.

   d. **False.** Atherosclerosis can occur in arteries of large or medium calibre. The presence of turbulent blood flow, smoking and high circulating LDL levels will all predispose to atherosclerosis.

   e. **False.** Lines of Zahn or other pale areas within a thrombus are caused by the presence of fibrin, which forms a network of insoluble fibrils.

2. a. **False.** In fact, the opposite is true. HDLs are involved in the transport of cholesterol from peripheral tissues to the liver. There is strong epidemiological evidence that high levels of HDL-cholesterol are associated with a reduced risk of heart disease and coronary artery atherosclerosis. High levels of low density lipoproteins (LDLs) are associated with heart disease.

   b. **True.** There is a relationship between high blood cholesterol levels and a high risk of coronary heart disease in Western countries and this is associated with diets which are high in saturated fat and cholesterol.

   c. **True.** The atherosclerotic plaque is composed of proliferating smooth muscle cells and macrophages, which also contain lipid. The fibrous cap of the plaque may be covered with normal endothelium or there may be ulceration and a superimposed thrombus.

   d. **True.** The atherosclerotic plaque is a proliferative and destructive lesion. The arterial wall becomes progressively less elastic and weaker as atherosclerosis progresses. Aneurysms commonly form as a result of this weakening. The most common site is the distal abdominal aorta.

   e. **True.** Superimposed thrombus is an important complication of atherosclerosis. It develops as a result of activation of the clotting cascade when plaque contents or blood vessel collagen are exposed to the blood. Platelet aggregation also occurs and triggers clotting. The resulting thrombus may propagate and cause occlusion of the vessel, for example in a coronary artery causing coronary thrombosis and myocardial infarction. Alternatively, the thrombus may break off and embolise to a distant vessel and cause occlusion there.

3. a. **False.** The lines of Zahn are pale stripes visible within a thrombus. In fact, they are caused by the fibrin meshwork within which red and white blood cells become trapped.

   b. **True.** An embolus is any fragment which breaks off and circulates in the blood to lodge at a distant site. Thrombi are a common cause of embolism. Less commonly, fragments of an atherosclerotic plaque, bacteria containing vegetations from a diseased heart valve, fat from a bone fracture or air can act as emboli.

   c. **True.** As the aneurysm enlarges because of the weakening of the aortic wall, there will be stasis of blood flow and thrombus forms in layers, gradually filling the sac. This thrombus may cause occlusion of blood flow to the legs via the iliac arteries or bits may break off and embolise to leg arteries, causing ischaemia of the foot.

   d. **True.** Thrombi commonly form over the surface of a myocardial infarction where the dead tissue is exposed to blood flowing through the heart chambers. A thrombus may propagate and build up within the ventricle. Again parts may break off and embolise to the brain via the carotid arteries, causing a stroke, or distally to other parts of the body such as the gut, spleen or legs.

   e. **False.** Cerebral infarction is caused by a reduction of blood supply to the brain. Embolism can be one cause of this but it is arterial embolism via the carotid arteries. Deep vein thrombosis occurs in the veins of the legs and embolises to the lungs. In very rare circumstances, a thrombus can embolise from the right atrium to the left atrium via a patent foramen ovale. This is known as paradoxical embolus where a thrombus originating in the deep veins embolises to the systemic circulation.

Case history answers

Case history 1

1. This woman has had a pulmonary embolus. A thrombus has detached itself from a deep vein in the pelvis or leg and embolised to a branch of the pulmonary artery. Because the lung has a dual blood supply from the pulmonary and bronchial arterial systems, infarction of the lung does not always occur with pulmonary embolism, unless the circulation is otherwise compromised, e.g. heart failure. The segment of infarcted lung has become necrotic and haemorrhagic. The pleural surface of the lung will be involved and give rise to the sharp pain that the patient experiences. Sometimes patients with pulmonary embolus and infarction develop haemoptysis (coughing up of blood) from the bleeding into the dead lung segment.

2. She has developed a thrombus in either a pelvic or deep leg vein. The factors of Virchow's triad, which determine whether a thrombus forms, are endothelial damage, increased coagulability or altered blood flow. In this case, pregnancy, especially with twins, may have led to stasis of blood in the pelvic veins and also an increase in the tendency to thrombose. Other well-known risk factors for this condition include myocardial infarction, immobility and the post-operative period.

3. Heparin is a quick-acting anticoagulant drug which acts as an antithrombin and inhibits factors IX and X. It is given subcutaneously or intravenously. Warfarin is an anticoagulant which is taken orally and takes about 24 hours to work. It inhibits the synthesis of vitamin K dependent clotting factors (II, VII, IX and X). Streptokinase is a fibrinolytic drug which is used in acute myocardial infarction and acts on thrombus to dissolve it and restore blood flow to the infarcted area of tissue.

Case history 2

1. The underlying pathological process is atherosclerosis and its complications. Gangrene of the large toe would be caused by occlusion of a digital artery, causing ischaemic infarction which then led to superadded infection with anaerobic organisms to produce gangrene. There are several possible causes of arterial occlusion; they include embolism, thrombotic occlusion and trauma. In this case, in an elderly heavy smoker, the most likely cause would be atheromatous embolism from the aorta. The patient had an abdominal aortic aneurysm containing thrombi, which is the most likely source of the embolism.

2. The main risk factors for atherosclerosis are being male, smoking, high ratio of low density lipoproteins to high density lipoproteins, diabetes and hypertension.

3. The complications of abdominal aortic aneurysm are:

   - atherosclerotic or thrombotic embolism to the lower limbs or to the gut or kidney
   - rupture with massive haemorrhage into the retroperitoneum and peritoneal cavity
   - severe atrophy of the lumbar vertebrae: this is thought to cause the classical backache experienced by many of these patients.

Short notes answers

With all the short notes questions, define the terms first and then explain the process and give some relevant examples.

1. An embolus is a mass of material which is carried in the bloodstream and can block a blood vessel. There are different types of embolus, but the most common is caused by a thrombus. Use pulmonary embolism from deep vein thrombosis as an example here. Other types of embolus include fat, air, amniotic fluid and atherosclerotic debris. Describe, using examples of these, the consequences of embolism in terms of infarction and the organs most likely to be affected.

2. Risk factors for coronary atherosclerosis are:

   - male sex
   - smoking
   - increasing age
   - hypertension
   - hyperlipidaemia
   - diabetes mellitus.

3. Infarction is an area of tissue death caused by a reduction in blood supply or venous drainage. Examples are myocardial infarction and venous infarction of testis. The reduced blood supply may be caused by embolism, thrombosis, vessel wall inflammation or arterial spasm. The consequences of infarction depend on the site and size of the blockage; infarction may affect the whole organ or may be segmental in nature.

Viva answers

1. A thrombus is:

   - a solid mass formed from blood constituents within the vascular system during life
   - attached to the vessel wall
   - made up of layers of platelets, white cells and red cells in a meshwork of fibrin (lines of Zahn).

   Predisposing factors are:

   - abnormal blood flow

- increased coagulability
- endothelial damage.

A clot is:

- a jelly-like mass which can occur after death or outside the body as well as within the body
- formed as an end product of the clotting cascade system

- formed via intrinsic and extrinsic pathway activity.

2. Modifiable risk factors for atherosclerosis are:

- smoking
- lack of exercise
- hyperlipidaemia (diet)
- diabetes mellitus.

The immune system 1

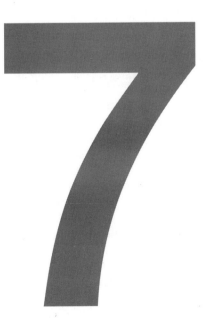

Chapter overview

The study of the immune system, immunology, is one of the most rapidly expanding and important areas of medicine. Diseases of the immune system, such as AIDS, have widespread and serious effects on the body which are seen in many branches of medicine. A sound knowledge of the basic principles of immunology is, therefore, important.

7.1 Natural defences and immunity

The human body is constantly bombarded from the outside world by potentially harmful substances and microorganisms. We have developed a sophisticated defence system to protect ourselves against these insults.

Innate immunity

Natural (innate) immunity is conferred by intact, tough physical barriers such as the skin, epithelial surfaces and basement membranes. Cellular barriers to infection include the alveolar macrophages, which can ingest inhaled particles, and neutrophils circulating in the blood. The acidity of the stomach and vaginal secretions provide hostile microenvironments which kill many organisms and the complement cascade is also a natural defence mechanism. These barriers are not specific against any one particular insult, but provide an effective first line of defence.

Adaptive immunity

Adaptive immunity is specific to the foreign substance which invokes it and becomes quicker and more intense with subsequent exposure to it. Thus the adaptive immune response 'remembers' previous challenges with the same substance and can mount a heightened and more rapid response. Adaptive immunity is only seen in higher vertebrates such as mammals.

Cells of the adaptive immune system

Lymphocytes are central to the adaptive immune response. There are two main types of lymphocyte, called B cells and T cells. Both these cell types possess membrane receptors which can bind to foreign material (**antigen**). This triggers a series of intracellular events in the lymphocyte which leads to its activation, multiplication and enhanced ability to destroy or neutralise the antigen.

Both types of lymphocyte are derived from precursor cells in the bone marrow. B cell maturation occurs in the bone marrow itself, whereas T cells migrate to the thymus for maturation. B and T cells have distinct functions, but they are interdependent and rely on cooperation with each other.

B cells

B cells have antibodies as their surface receptors. Once the appropriate antigen binds to the antibody, activation of the B cell occurs. Ultimately the B cell develops into a plasma cell which synthesises and secretes large amounts of the antibody into the extracellular fluid, allowing disposal of the antigen. This process is known as **humoral immunity.**

T cells

These have a surface antigen recognition system known as the T cell receptor, which is similar to the antibody molecule. There are discrete subsets of T cells which, when triggered by antigen-receptor binding, have functions as diverse as killing cells, coordinating B and T cell responses and stopping the immune response. T cells are particularly involved with the immune response to intracellular organisms (e.g. viruses and special bacteria such as *Mycobacterium tuberculosis*). This process is known as **cellular immunity.**

Organisation of the adaptive immune system

In order to optimise the combined functions of surveillance of the body's tissues for antigen and production of a coordinated immune response, the cells of the adaptive immune response are organised into structured lymphoid tissues (lymph nodes, tonsils, thymus and spleen). Lymphoid tissue is also found in the gut (Peyer's patches) and the bone marrow.

The bone marrow and the thymus are sometimes known as primary lymphoid organs, where lymphocytes are produced and mature, whereas the peripheral lymph nodes and other lymphoid sites are called secondary organs, where lymphocytes live and recognise antigens and initiate the immune response.

There are similarities in the structure of many of the lymphoid tissues (e.g. lymph node, Fig. 17). In general, B cells are found and proliferate in discrete nodular structures known as lymphoid follicles. These follicles are often surrounded by a sea of T lymphocytes (admixed with other cells of the immune response and small blood or lymphatic channels). Lymphocytes can circulate via the lymphatics and bloodstream between lymphoid organs.

Properties of the immune response

Specificity

The response is specific: most antigens are foreign macromolecules or microbes and these are made up of large numbers of differently shaped structural components (usually proteins or carbohydrates). Some of these components, called the **antigenic determinants,** will be

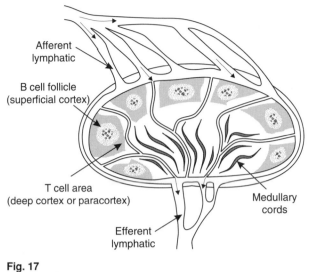

Fig. 17
Lymph node structure.

Afferent lymphatic

B cell follicle (superficial cortex)

T cell area (deep cortex or paracortex)

Efferent lymphatic

Medullary cords

recognised by a receptor on the membrane of one or a restricted number of lymphocytes. Only these few lymphocytes can, therefore, initially respond to the foreign substance.

Memory

The immune response has memory. Exposure to a previously encountered antigen results in a quicker and larger response. This is at least in part through the generation of memory cells during the first challenge with antigen. Memory cells have the antigen receptor on their surface and on a subsequent occasion can proliferate quickly to mount a response.

Diversity

The response is diverse. The number of different antigen-specific lymphocytes is vast. We have millions of lymphocytes, each bearing a receptor recognising a slightly different shaped or structured antigenic determinant. When exposed to a particular antigen, e.g. a bacterium, the lymphocyte with the appropriate receptor is selected from this vast available pool and stimulated to multiply. This process is called **clonal selection.**

The diversity of the system results from the variability in the structure of the lymphocyte surface receptor. The basic structure of the T cell receptor and the immunoglobulin molecule are similar, both being members of the immunoglobulin 'superfamily'. The molecular mechanisms which enable the lymphocytes to generate such diverse receptors is now beginning to be understood. Central to the process is the phenomenon of random rearrangement of a small number of genes within the cell allowing the generation of many different receptors. The details of the genetic mechanisms underlying the generation of antibody diversity (particularly in relation to the marked heterogeneity of the variable regions) are beyond the scope of this book. However, multiple mechanisms are used to generate variable region diversity, both in antibody molecules

and in the T cell receptor. Molecular techniques such as Southern blot analysis (see Ch. 2) have shown that immunoglobulin gene-containing DNA fragments are of a different size in B cells and cells that do not produce antibody. This can be explained by the genes being far apart in 'ordinary' cells, but close together in B cells. B cells must therefore be able to rearrange these genes during their development. This is done in a precise order (e.g. the first rearrangement involves the heavy chains, etc.).

Recognition of self

The immune system can distinguish between self and non-self. Thus under normal circumstances, lymphocytes recognise and respond to molecules that they perceive as foreign but apparently ignore the millions of potential antigens present in normal human tissues and organs. This non-response to our own tissues by our own lymphocytes is known as **tolerance** and is partly achieved by the early deletion (by apoptosis) of potentially self-reacting cells. It is only when cells reacting with self escape from control measures that **autoimmune** disease occurs and our own tissues become damaged and destroyed.

7.2 **Humoral immunity**

The B cell response

Antibodies are synthesised by B cells; they are then secreted into the tissue fluids for combination with antigen or are inserted into the B cell membrane to act as a receptor. If a human is exposed to a number of antigens (or even a single antigen), a number of B cells may each recognise a different component of the antigen by means of their surface antibody (immunoglobulin) receptor. The proliferation of different B cells with different antibodies being produced by the resultant plasma cells is called a **polyclonal response**.

Occasionally, a **monoclonal response** may occur. The classical naturally occurring example of this is when a patient suffers from an abnormal proliferation of a single B cell (in effect a cancer of the B cell), resulting in the production of millions of only one type of plasma cell and thus one single type of antibody. This malignant proliferation of plasma cells is known as multiple myeloma. Monoclonal antibodies can also be manufactured in the laboratory and have an important role in both investigative and clinical medicine (see Chapter 2).

Antibody structure

The basic structure of an antibody is shown in Figure 18. In its simplest form, an antibody is composed of two identical light chains and two identical heavy chains. The molecular weight is about 150 000. The light chains are joined to the heavy chains and the heavy chains to each other by covalent disulphide bonds. Overall, the antibody molecule has a 'Y' shape, with movement of

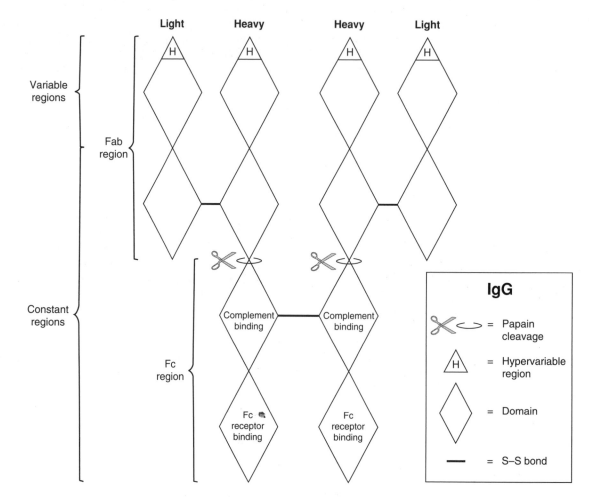

Fig. 18
The basic structure of an antibody (immunoglobulin).

the arms possible at the hinge. The end of the arms are actually where antigen binding occurs. Light chains and heavy chains can be further subdivided into **domains**, each approximately 110 amino acid residues long. There are four domains per heavy chain and two per light chain. The domains fulfil a common role in different antibodies. Biochemical analysis of these domains has shown that the amino acid sequence in the N-terminal domain of both the light and heavy chains is very variable — the so called **variable region** — and it is here that antigen binding occurs. The remaining domains are relatively constant — the **constant regions**.

There are different classes of antibody with different functions (Table 8), but all are based on the simple prototype.

Table 8 Classes and functions of antibodies

Antibody class	Functions
IgM	First class of antibody produced before IgG supervenes Pentamer with 10 antigen-binding sites Intravascular: cannot cross placenta Activates complement and agglutinates foreign substances
IgG	Four subclasses Can attach to phagocytic cells via Fc fragment (opsonisation) Found in tissues and can cross placenta Activates complement
IgA	Main antibody in secretions and excretions and in urine and gut contents Two subclasses: can dimerise (MW 320 000) and have a secretory piece added — this prevents digestion Stops microbes entering tissues from external surfaces
IgE	Involved in acute allergic reaction (type 1 hypersensitivity) Involved in defence against parasites
IgD	Found on the surface of B lymphocytes (?)Regulatory and recognition molecule

The antibody response

Certain antigens, e.g. large polysaccharides, can trigger antibody production directly. Others, including most proteins, require T cells — T helper cells (CD4+) — to assist in triggering antibody production. T helper cells secrete a vast array of cytokines that drive the differentiation of B cells into antibody-secreting plasma cells.

There is a significant difference between the response to antigen of previously unstimulated B cells (the **primary** antibody response) and the response of memory B cells which have been produced during a previous encounter with the same antigen (the **secondary** antibody response). The primary response takes longer and usually involves the production of IgM. The secondary response is faster and IgG predominates. The secondary reaction only occurs with T cell-dependent protein antigens. The processes occurring in the B cell to achieve a response to antigen are shown in Figures 19 and 20.

The fate of antigen–antibody immune complexes

We are constantly being challenged by antigens and the formation of small numbers of antigen–antibody (immune) complexes is a normal event. When we mount an antibody response to a bacterial infection, vast numbers of immune complexes are formed as antibody binds to and neutralises bacterial antigens.

The disposal of immune complexes is important since, potentially, they can lodge in blood vessel walls and cause damage by activating complement and initiating an inflammatory reaction. In fact, components of the complement cascade can interfere with immune complex formation by binding to immunoglobulin and hindering the interaction with antigen, or by facilitating disposal of the complexes by macrophage-derived phagocytes in various tissues.

Antigen-presenting cells

Macrophages and antigen presenting cells (APC) play a part in both natural and specific immunity. They phagocytose, process and present antigens to B cells and T cells, in association with MHC class II molecules. They also produce cytokines and other factors which coordinate and amplify the immune response. Examples of APC include Kupffer cells of the liver, Langerhans' cells of the skin and dendritic cells of the B cell follicle.

7.3 Cellular immunity

T cell-mediated immunity

T cells, which mediate the cellular immune response, have two major functions:

- recognition and attack of cell surface antigens
- regulation of the T and B cells in the immune response.

There are several subclasses of T cells, which can be recognised immunohistochemically by antibodies to different surface protein markers; these markers exist as clusters of antigens. One classification system is known as cluster differentiation and cells are given CD numbers to describe their surface antigen. The subclasses also have different functional characteristics (Table 9). CD4+ T helper cells (T_H), which represent about 60% of the total T cell number, can only recognise antigen when it is presented together with antigen of the MHC (major histocompatibility complex) class II antigen. CD8+ cells can only recognise antigen when presented with class I MHC antigen. This is known as restriction: a response can only be mounted against an antigen that is presented with the correct MHC molecule.

T helper cells are an important part of the defence against extracellular antigens. Class II antigens display a sample of extracellular proteins that have been endocytosed. Class II antigens are only found on antigen-presenting cells (APC), activated macrophages, B cells and some T cells.

Class I antigens are found on all nucleated cells and platelets. Class I antigens display a sample of the intracellular protein content; this can stimulate the CD8+ cytotoxic T cells (T_C) to destroy such cells displaying foreign protein, e.g. as a result of viral infection.

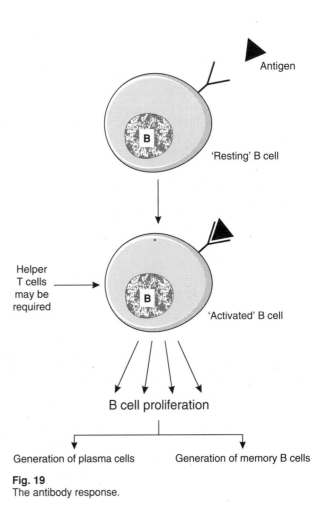

Fig. 19
The antibody response.

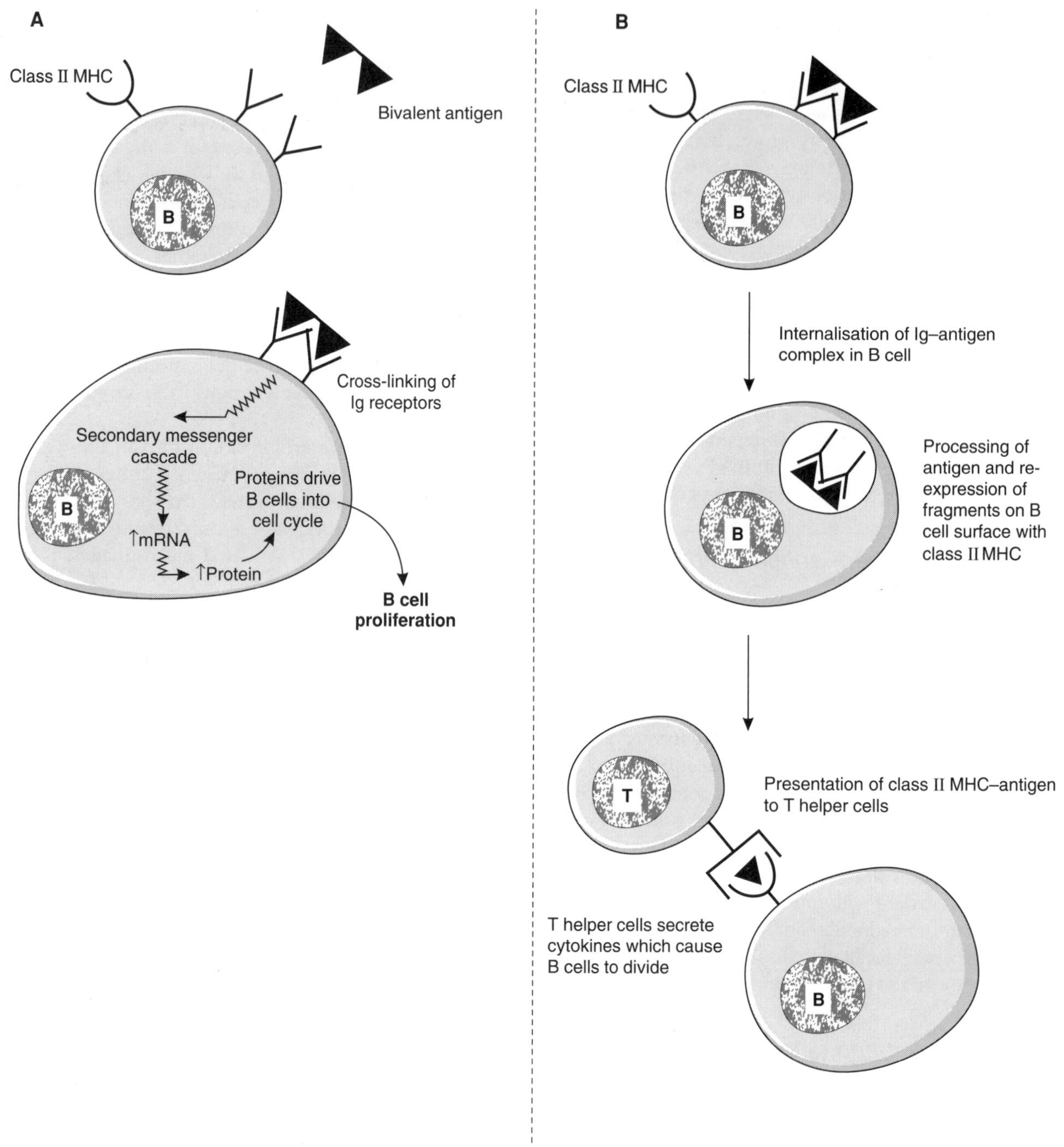

A

Class II MHC

Bivalent antigen

B

Cross-linking of
Ig receptors

Secondary messenger
cascade

↑mRNA

Proteins drive
B cells into
cell cycle

B

↑Protein

**B cell
proliferation**

B

Class II MHC

B

Internalisation of Ig–antigen
complex in B cell

B

Processing of
antigen and re-
expression of
fragments on B
cell surface with
class II MHC

T

Presentation of class II MHC–antigen
to T helper cells

T helper cells secrete
cytokines which cause
B cells to divide

B

Fig. 20
How antigens trigger B cells to produce antibody.

Table 9 T lymphocyte subsets

T cell subset	Function	CD status	MHC requirement
Helper/inducer (T_H)	Earliest response to antigen on APC, which facilitates B + T cell responses	CD4+, CD8-	II
Delayed hypersensitivity (T_D)	On contact with antigen releases cytokines and recruits macrophages	CD4+; CD8-	II
Cytotoxic (T_C)	Kills cells of transplants and any cell showing abnormal surface antigens	CD4-, CD8+	I
Suppressor (T_S)	Suppresses immune response, particularly against self	CD4-, CD8+	I

The restriction of class II expression means that CD4$^+$ T helper cells, which trigger many of the immune responses, can only be activated by a limited number of cell types. If T helper cells were activated by class I antigens found on all nucleated cells, the immune response would be continuously triggered.

How do T cells attack antigen?

T cell attack on antigen is mainly seen when cells have been infected by viruses, or in transplant rejection and skin reactions to certain chemicals. Cytotoxic T cells (T$_C$) and delayed hypersensitivity cells (T$_D$) are the main T cells involved.

Cytotoxic T cells

Cytotoxic T cells kill virus-infected cells, thus stopping the manufacture and spread of viral particles. The viral antigen (as an intracellular protein) is displayed on the host cell surface in association with class I antigen. The infected cell is in effect alerting the cytotoxic T cell, which kills the cell by making it undergo apoptosis or by inserting a doughnut-shaped protein (perforin) into the cell membrane. The cell cytoplasm then 'bleeds' out through the hole.

Delayed hypersensitivity T cells

These are important in mycobacterial infections (tuberculosis). In individuals previously exposed to and infected by tuberculosis, an intracutaneous injection of an extract of the TB organism causes recruitment of circulating T cells with specificities against the TB antigen. The delayed hypersensitivity T helper cells release soluble protein molecules (cytokines and lymphokines) which attract macrophages to the site of infection. Macrophages are also activated, allowing intracellular killing of the organism.

During the process of aggregation and activation of macrophages, some may change their shape and resemble epithelial cells (so called epithelioid macrophages) and others may fuse together to form giant cells. These aggregates of macrophages are called granulomas (see p. 83).

Suppressor T cells

These cells function to inhibit (de-activate) the immune response. Relatively little is known about how they do this. They may not require processing and display of antigen by antigen-presenting cells and, therefore, may not be MHC restricted, despite being CD8$^+$. They probably perform their suppressor functions by secreting proteins (inhibitory cytokines) which stop cell activation or proliferation or directly cause cell death by lysis.

7.4 Other components of the immune response

Cytokines

These are soluble, polypeptide molecules, produced by cells involved in the immune response, which act as messengers between the cells. This allows communication between the cells and coordination of the complex chain of events which occurs in response to antigen.

Examples of cytokines include **interleukins**, which are involved in lymphocyte proliferation and differentiation, **interferons**, which protect against viral infection, and **colony-stimulating factors**, which regulate the production of bone marrow blood cells.

The major histocompatibility complex (MHC)

The MHC system occurs in all vertebrates and is the major system distinguishing self and non-self. The human MHC system is known as the humanleucocyte antigen (HLA) system. The HLA system is a large group of genes found on the short arm of chromosome 6. It has been known for some time that these genes code for cell surface glycoproteins and initially it was thought that they were used only in transplant rejection. It is now known that they are important in many cell-mediated immunological reactions and help lymphocytes to identify cells with which they need to interact.

The six loci that code for these cell surface glycoproteins are known as *DP, DQ, DR* (class II genes producing class II antigens) and *A, B* and *C* (class I genes/antigens) (Table 10). At each of these loci, there are numerous possible alleles (versions of the gene). Therefore, the number of possible combinations on both chromosomes is astronomical.

Class I antigens are transmembrane glycoproteins and consist of two polypeptide chains which grip peptide fragments to be presented to cytotoxic T cells (CD8$^+$). If the peptide is not a normal part of the cell, such as a viral protein, it is recognised and the cell destroyed.

Class II MHC molecules are also composed of two polypeptide chains spanning the cell membrane. The

Table 10 Major histocompatibility antigens[a]

Class	Chromosome location	Number of molecules	Cell location
I	6	3 (HLA-A, B, C)	All nucleated cells
II	6	3 (HLA-DP, DQ, DR)	Antigen-presenting cells

[a] Each of the class I and class II molecules is polymorphic (has many variants). One person can only exhibit two variants of each molecule, one coded by each parent.

main function of these molecules is to present foreign antigens to CD4$^+$ T helper cells.

Most nucleated cells display class I antigens, but only a few, specialised cells such as dendritic cells, macrophages and Langerhan's cells (i.e. APCs), display class II. Class II antigens are very potent at stimulating T cell proliferation.

Since the advent of tissue typing, it has been found that some diseases are common in people with a particular type or combination of types of HLA. Perhaps the best known example is the arthritic disease ankylosing spondylitis where the *HLA B27* allele is found about 20 times more commonly in patients than in non-sufferers.

Complement

The complement system is an enzymatic cascade which can be activated by antibody (classical pathway) or anti-gen (alternate pathway) or both. Complement proteins are made in the liver and are numbered 1–9.

Killer cells

This special type of (non B, non T) lymphocyte has receptors for the Fc portion of IgG on its surface and therefore can bind to IgG-coated cells. The killer cell then destroys the coated cell by insertion of perforin channels. This type of killing is called antibody-dependent cell-mediated cytotoxicity.

7.5 Summary

All the components discussed in this chapter have specific roles in the immune response and are interlinked in their functions and requirements for activation (Table 11 and Fig. 21).

Table 11 The immune response: principal players and their functions

Component	Function
B lymphocytes	Recognition of antigen Presentation of antigenic peptides to CD4 T cells Secretion of antibody
CD4 T helper lymphocytes	Recognition of antigens on MHC class II cells after endocytosis and processing Promoting local inflammation by recruitment and activation of macrophages Helping T and/or B cell responses
CD8 T cytotoxic lymphocytes	Recognition of intracellular antigens presented on MHC class I cells after cytosolic processing Killing cells which present abnormal proteins in class I MHC
Macrophages	Phagocytosis and destruction of microbes, dead cells and tissue debris, promoted by coatings of antibody and complement Walling off infection in granulomas Presentation of antigens to CD4$^+$ cells
Antibodies	Capture of antigen by B cells Neutralising toxins and microbial invaders Ear-marking microbes and abnormal body cells for destruction by complement and effector cells
Cytokines	Control of cellular activities

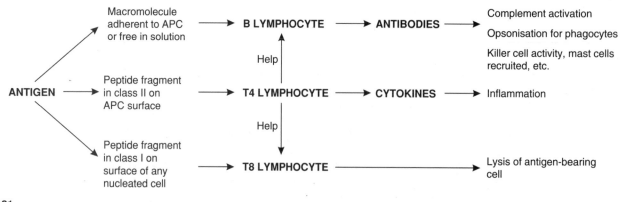

Fig. 21
Overview of the immune response

Self-assessment: questions

Multiple choice questions

1. The following are correctly paired:
   a. IgG — cannot cross placenta
   b. CD8 — class II MHC
   c. IgM — complement activation
   d. B cells — cell-mediated immunity
   e. Interleukin-1 (IL-1) — fever

2. The following statements are true:
   a. Dendritic cells and Langerhans' cells can present antigen
   b. IgD is found in secretions such as tears and sweat
   c. CD3 is found on T cells
   d. Proliferation of cytotoxic (CD8$^+$) T cells usually requires the presence of helper (CD4$^+$) cells
   e. In humans, the genes for the MHC system are found on chromosome 7

Case history

A 10-year-old girl develops a sore throat. A throat swab grows a streptococcus bacterium. During the course of her illness, she is noted by her GP to have enlarged neck lymph nodes.

1. What changes would you expect to see in this girl's lymph nodes?
2. How might this differ if the infection was viral?

Despite prompt treatment with antibiotics, the sore throat takes quite a few days to resolve. Two weeks after her throat problems have gone, she notices that her urine is bloodstained and she begins to feel generally unwell.

3. How might this second illness relate to her sore throat?
4. What potential immune-mediated problems are associated with streptococcal sore throat?

Essay questions

1. Describe the MHC (major histocompatibility complex) system. What is the normal function of this system?
2. Describe the key features of the T cell-dependent antibody response. When might T cell-independent B cell responses occur?
3. Discuss the structure and function of IgG. What similarities are there between antibody molecules and the T cell receptor?

Viva questions

Discuss:

1. Humoral versus cell-mediated immunity
2. Cytokines/interleukins
3. Antigen-presenting cells
4. MHC
5. CD molecules
6. Antibody diversity
7. Innate versus adaptive immunity.

Self-assessment: answers

Multiple choice answers

1. a. **False.** IgG can cross the placenta; it is IgM that cannot. IgM is the first antibody to be produced in the immune response. This is quickly superceded by IgG. If IgM antibodies to a particular organism are present within the fetal circulation, this indicates that it is the fetus itself which is infected and mounting an immune response. IgG antibodies could be maternal in origin.
   b. **False.** CD4+ (helper) T cells recognise antigen in association with class II MHC molecules. CD8+ (cytotoxic) T cells use class I molecules.
   c. **True.** IgM is very efficient at complement activation.
   d. **False.** Cell-mediated immunity centres on cytotoxic T cell responses and involves T cell and macrophage interaction. Natural killer (NK) cells are also involved. These are a class of lymphocyte which in vitro can kill tumour cells without prior antigen stimulation. Their in vivo function is not completely known. Both B cells and T cells are required for the humoral immune response.
   e. **True.** Fever (high temperature, pyrexia) is caused by a number of cytokines, including interleukin-1 (see viva answer 2).

2. a. **True.** There are a large number of antigen-presenting cells (APCs). Classical APCs include dendritic cells in lymph nodes, skin Langerhan's cells and macrophages. In addition, B cells can present antigen to, and control the activation of, T cells.
   b. **False.** IgA is found in secretions.
   c. **True.** There are numerous CD molecules on the surface of lymphocytes, macrophages and APCs. The structure and function of many of these protein molecules are now well characterised. CD4 and CD8 are perhaps the best known. CD3 is found on all T cells associated with the T cell receptor.
   d. **True.** The function of the cytotoxic (CD8+) T cell is to destroy viral-infected cells, recognised by the association of class I MHC molecules with viral antigens on the surface of the infected cell. In order to proliferate, the CD8+ cell requires stimulation by cytokines (IL-2) from CD4+ T helper cells.
   e. **False.** The genes of the human MHC (known as the HLA) are found on the short arm of chromosome 6. There are two sets of genes (class I and class II) and each contains three loci. Each locus has a large number of alleles coding for MHC antigens.

Case history answer

1. Bacterial infections tend to elicit a strong humoral (antibody) immune response. The local lymph nodes draining the site of infection will be stimulated to produce plasma cells. In a normal lymph node, B cell areas are found in the outer cortex and are known as follicles — densely packed aggregates of cells. When B cell production is stimulated, these follicles acquire a germinal centre. Transformation of B cells occurs in germinal centres with the production of numerous memory cells. B cells differentiate into plasma cells in the cortical areas deep to and between the follicles — the paracortex. Plasma cells then enter the medullary vascular system (medullary cords) and produce antibody as they leave in the efferent lymphatics, draining the site of infection. The local lymph nodes will have large cortical follicles with prominent germinal centres.

2. In contrast, viral infections generally stimulate a T cell response — cytotoxic T cells (CD8+) can recognise and destroy infected cells if the viral antigen is displayed on the cell's surface in association with a class I MHC molecule. The T cell areas of the lymph node are found in the paracortex and massive expansion of this region can occur during viral infections — the B cell follicles may be relatively inconspicuous.

3. Streptococcal antigen combined with antibody has deposited in her kidneys causing them to function abnormally.

   There are a variety of consequences when antigen and antibody combine to form an immune complex. Antibodies may bind to bacteria, preventing them from entering cells and thus negating their effects. Complement may be activated and the antigen destroyed. If the immune complex evades phagocytic clearance mechanisms and persists in the circulation, it may deposit in organs, evoking an inflammatory reaction which causes damage (e.g. kidney, joints, skin). In this case, the immune complexes have deposited in the renal glomerulus and the inflammatory reaction and cell proliferation induced causes the glomerulus to malfunction and become leaky. Blood can then be found in the urine (haematuria). Fortunately, in most cases, once the inflammatory response has died down, normal kidney function is restored. The delay in onset of the problem is a result of the time taken to produce large amounts of antibody.

4. One important condition which occurs after a streptococcal infection is rheumatic fever. In this disease, now very rare in USA, Canada and Europe, antibodies produced against streptococcal antigens

cross-react with antigens in the patient's own tissues. The heart is often affected and the inflammatory damage may lead to fibrosis and distortion of the valves. This can lead to heart failure and death if the valve is not replaced.

Essay answers

1. The MHC system in humans is known as the human leucocyte system (HLA). It is a large group of genes, found on the short arm of chromosome 6 in humans, and is responsible for the body's ability to distinguish self from non-self and enabling defence against foreign agents such as bacteria and viruses (see Table 11).
2. Many antigens, including most proteins, can only trigger antibody production with the help of T cells — T helper (CD4$^+$) cells. These cells secrete cytokines that stimulate the production of antibody- secreting plasma cells from B cells. T cell-independent B cell responses: in rare instances, B cells can be stimulated by antigen directly, without the requirement for T cell help. This occurs with large antigens, which often have repeating units, i.e. are 'polymeric'.
3. The immunoglobulin molecule and the T cell receptor share many common features and are part of an 'immunoglobulin superfamily'. All the members of this group are made up of polypeptide chains with domains. The T cell receptor contains alpha and beta or gamma and delta chains. It confers upon the T cell (CD4$^+$ or CD8$^+$) specificity for both antigen and MHC. The post-stimulus response of the T cell is dependent on other surface molecules such as CD3. Gene rearrangement occurs during production of the T cell receptor in a similar manner to immunoglobulin production.

Viva answers

Any of these topics may come up in a viva or short notes question. Because immunology is complicated and there are numerous facts to remember, it is a good idea to be able to define all the basic terms. Go through this chapter and look in the glossary (p. 119) and find the definitions. As with all other areas of pathology, have some examples to which you can refer. For example, when defining the appearances, type and function of antigen-presenting cells, use the dendritic cells of the lymph node (or spleen) as an example. Remember an APC must be able to i) endocytose and process macromolecules and ii) express MHC Class II. It is also very important to be able to demonstrate that you understand how the different components of the immune system interact. Practise a simple overview diagram or algorithm that will help you to do this. You should be able to give a definition for each of these topics or processes. In addition, the examiners will want to be sure that you know how they may link together within the immune system.

1. The main points to cover are:
   - B cells and T cells: origin and main functions
   - B cells produce antibody to neutralise antigen
   - T cells (CD8$^+$) may directly kill antigen-bearing cells or produce cytokines (CD4$^+$) which enhance the inflammatory reaction
   - B and T cells are interdependent
   - Examples of immunosuppression lack of T or B cells, e.g. SCID or AIDS (see next chapter).

   This is a very broad topic and you should be able to give a broad overview of the topic. The examiners will inevitably focus on details at any point.

2. Define both. Cytokines are regulatory proteins concerned with a variety of biological processes: cell growth, cell activation, inflammation, immunity, and tissue repair. An example is interferons: antiviral cytokines produced by leucocytes in response to viral infection. Interleukins are a family of molecules produced mainly by leucocytes and form a class of cytokines.

   Interferon:
   - produced by macrophages
   - cell targets: lymphocytes, monocytes, tissue cells
   - main actions: immunuregulation (increases MHCI expression), antiviral action.

   Interleukin 1:
   - produced by: lymphocytes, monocytes/macrophages, tissue cells, endothelium
   - cell targets: endothelium, hypothalmus, T + B cells
   - main actions: immunoregulation, inflammation, fever.

   Interleukin 2:

   'T cellgrowth factor'
   - produced by T cells (Mainly CD4$^+$)
   - cell targets: T + B cells, monocytes
   - main actions: autocrine, paracrine, proliferation, activation.

   Other interleukins have a variety of functions and interactions. Details of these are not necessary but can be obtained from more detailed immunology textbooks.

3. Define the nature and function of antigen-presenting cells. Outline their structural characteristics, e.g. large surface area for antigen presentation. Give examples: dendritic cells in lymph nodes, Langerhan's cells in skin.

4. See the answer to essay question 1 and Table 11.

5. Cluster differentiation (CD) molecules are cell surface molecules of leucocytes, platelets and other

cells. They can be identified by binding with monoclonal or polyclonal antibodies and are used to differentiate different cell populations or sub-populations. Examples are CD8$^+$ and CD4$^+$ T lymphocytes.

6. Read the explanation of antibody diversity earlier in this chapter. It is important to have a concept of why this is important in relation to the immune system:

how it is brought about; the role of gene rearrangements in achieving the diversity of T and B cell receptors.

7. Innate immunity comprises the natural defence mechanisms, e.g. skin, tears, etc. Adaptive immunity consists of specific immune responses to a certain foreign macromolecule (antigen) — B cells, T cells, etc.

The immune system 2

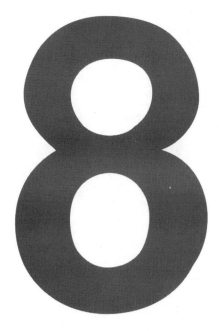

Chapter overview

The normal immune system is designed to enable the body to deal with foreign substances which would cause damage and disease. However, sometimes the immune reaction has undesirable and damaging effects on its own tissues. This is known as immunological injury and can arise from **hypersensitivity** reactions, where the host tissue is secondarily destroyed during an immune response, or by the process of **autoimmunity**, where the immune system fails to distinguish between self and non-self antigens.

8.1 Hypersensitivity

Hypersensitivity is a process whereby the host's tissue is injured during an immune response to a foreign antigen. When this process becomes non-physiological (i.e. uncontrolled), 'hypersensitivity diseases' occur.

Type I hypersensitivity

In type I hypersensitivity, the immune reaction is immediate and triggers the release of substances that cause blood vessels to leak and cause smooth muscle contraction. The reaction can be localised or generalised.

Localised reactions

The most common examples of localised type I hypersensitivity reactions are asthma, hay fever and urticaria. In susceptible, sensitised individuals, exposure to antigen (allergen) results in an immediate and acute immune response which is mediated by IgE. It is not known why IgE is the antibody produced in this situation. The reaction can be triggered by substances which are commonly found all around us. For example asthma can be triggered by house dust or animal proteins, and hay fever can be caused by pollen.

Generalised reactions

Rarely, antigens enter the bloodstream of a sensitised individual and bind to IgE on circulating basophils. This can lead to a severe reaction known as **anaphylaxis** in which there is acute bronchospasm, circulatory collapse as a result of peripheral vasodilatation, shock and even death. This may happen to people who are sensitised to penicillin or bee stings.

Sequence of events

This is the same in both localised and generalised immediate hypersensitivity reactions. In sensitised people, IgE is bound to the surface of tissue mast cells and basophils, which have specific receptors for the Fc portion of the antibody, leaving the antigen-binding sites free to link with antigen. This binding has high affinity. After antigen and IgE have linked together, there follows an increase in membrane permeability to calcium with activation of enzymes including adenylyl cyclase. This leads to **degranulation of mast cells**, which release histamine, a powerful vasodilator and constrictor of smooth muscle, and an eosinophil chemotactic factor (Table 12). Degranulation of mast cells can be caused by substances other than IgE, e.g. drugs such as morphine.

Independent of the granule system, there is local release of bioactive lipids, which are synthesised and produced by the activated mast cells in the vicinity. These substances include leukotrienes, including substance previously known as the slow releasing substance of anaphylaxis (SRS-A), and some prostaglandins (see Table 12). These also cause smooth muscle constriction and may be very important in the pathogenesis of asthma.

Type II hypersensitivity reaction

In type II hypersensitivity reactions, antibody binds directly to tissues: antibodies are directed against and bind with normal or altered components on the cell surface which they recognise as non-self. This causes cell damage by complement activation and lysis or by binding to macrophages and phagocytosis. Important examples of such reactions are:

- incompatible blood transfusion reaction
- haemolytic disease of the newborn.

Incompatible blood transfusion reaction

Antibodies against rhesus or ABO blood group antigen, bind directly on the surface of the blood cells, causing haemolysis.

Table 12 Properties of mast cells

	Action
Substances found in mast cell granules	
Eosinophil and neutrophil chemotactic factors	Chemotaxis
Histamine	Vasodilatation, increased permeability
Heparin	Late phase reactions
Trypsin	Late phase reactions
Substances made by mast cells during response	
Leukotrienes	Chemotaxis, smooth muscle contraction
Prostaglandins	Vasodilatation, smooth muscle contraction
Platelet-activating factor	Platelet aggregation, smooth muscle contraction, increased permeability

Haemolytic disease of the newborn

Rhesus (Rh) blood group antigens are present in about 85% of people (rhesus positive); the remainder of the population are rhesus negative. Rhesus antigen is inherited through a dominant gene (D) so that rhesus-positive individuals can be homozygous (DD) or heterozygous (Dd). Haemolytic disease of the newborn may arise if a rhesus-negative mother carries a rhesus-positive fetus. When fetal red cells enter the maternal circulation (usually at delivery), maternal antibodies against fetal rhesus antigen will be produced. The first rhesus-positive baby from a rhesus-negative mother is usually normal, but subsequent babies from a sensitised mother will develop progressively more severe haemolysis. The disease can be prevented by injecting the mother with IgG rhesus antibody immediately after delivery to 'mop up' any fetal cells and prevent her producing natural antibody.

Type III hypersensitivity

In type III hypersensitivity, antibodies react with antigens forming antigen–antibody complexes that can be deposited either locally or at a distant site. The antigen–antibody (immune) complexes cause tissue damage when they are deposited, usually in blood vessel walls, where they induce an inflammatory reaction as a result of complement activation and infiltration by neutrophils.

Localised immune complex disease (Arthus reaction)

The Arthus reaction is an example of immune complex damage following injection of an antigen into the skin of an individual with high levels of preformed antibody. Within 2–8 hours, a haemorrhagic oedematous reaction occurs. After 12–24 hours, skin necrosis occurs as a result of localised vasculitis (inflammation of vessels causing necrosis of the wall) from local immune complex deposition. Histologically there is an acute inflammatory reaction with numerous neutrophils.

Systemic immune complex disease

When an antigen first stimulates the formation of antibody, there is antigen excess. As levels of antibody rise, antigen/antibody equivalence occurs and as antigen is removed, there is a relative excess of antibody in the circulation. Small soluble immune complexes are formed when there is antigen excess. They are not easily phagocytosed and may deposit out into the walls of blood vessels in the kidney (glomerulus), heart, joints and skin. Here they activate complement and cause tissue damage. Large harmless immune complexes are formed when there is antigen/antibody equivalence or antibody excess and these are readily cleared from the circulation by macrophage phagocytosis.

There are various clinical situations in which systemic immune complexes can form and cause disease:

Systemic lupus erythematosus

Definition. Chronic illness with fluctuating activity. Multisystem involvement especially skin, joints, kidneys and serosal surfaces.

Age/sex. Young to middle-aged females.

Cause. Most cases are spontaneous and probably mediated by polyclonal B cell hyperactivity with autoantibody production and immune complex formation. Most important autoantibodies are antinuclear (anti-double-stranded DNA antibodies); this is diagnostic of the disease. Some cases occur in patients on drugs (hydralazine). The tissue injury is caused by a type 3 hypersensitivity reaction.

Pathological processes. The main pathological changes and their resulting symptoms are:
- vasculitis (inflammation of vessels) with necrosis: rashes, muscle weakness
- glomerulonephritis: haematuria, proteinuria, renal failure
- synovitis: arthritis
- pleuritis, lung inflammation: chest pain, breathlessness
- pericarditis, endocarditis: chest pain, heart failure

Clinical course. Very varied. A few patients die rapidly with heart/renal failure. Most have a chronic illness requiring repeated courses of immunosuppressive drugs.

- infection: e.g. post-streptococcal glomerulonephritis
- autoimmune disease, e.g. systemic lupus erythematosus (see the box above).

Type IV hypersensitivity

Type IV hypersensitivity is a delayed reaction characterised by the involvement of T lymphocytes. The response is usually to viruses, fungi, protozoans and mycobacteria, but it is also seen in transplanted organs. Antibodies are not involved. It takes time for primed T cells to react and hence there is a delay of at least 12 hours before the reaction can be seen. The prototype of this reaction is the tuberculin test. If a small amount of protein derived from tubercle bacilli is injected into the skin of a non-immune person, there will be no reaction. However, in people who have already had tuberculosis (TB) or been immunised with BCG (derived from TB) and, therefore, have primed T cells, an area of reddening develops in 12 hours. The reaction is maximal at 1 week and histologically the tissue at the reaction site shows a granuloma, which is an accumulation of lymphocytes, macrophages and epithelioid cells (transformed macrophages). Macrophages often fuse together to form giant cells.

At the first encounter with the tubercle bacillus, CD4+ T cells recognise antigen when it is presented with class II MHC molecules on antigen-presenting cells (APCs).

Memory T cells are then formed. On re-encountering the antigen, sensitised T cells react with antigen on the APC surface, become stimulated to produce lymphokines (e.g. interleukin-2) which in turn activate CD8⁺ T cells and recruit macrophages into the area. Interleukin-1 from macrophages increases T cell proliferation and promotes the release of acute phase reactants, which are important in fever production.

8.2 Autoimmune disease

Patients with autoimmune disease have antibodies against their own tissues (autoantibodies) in their blood. Autoimmune disease can affect one particular cell type, one organ system or many systems of the body (multi-system disease). The exact mechanism by which the body's immune system is triggered to attack itself is not known. It is possible that cross-reaction of an antibody produced against a foreign antigen (e.g. bacterium) with a normal tissue antigen occurs (rheumatic heart disease) or that tissue antigens can be altered by drugs. Marked changes in MHC expression occur, with both increased expression and de novo expression of class II in previously negative cell types (see the box below). In addition, abnormalities in the regulation of T and B lymphocyte function have also been implicated. The classical example of a multi-system, autoimmune disease is systemic lupus erythematosus. Another is rheumatoid disease; the main features are shown in the box, right.

8.3 Transplantation

Since the late 1960s, organ transplantation has become commonplace. Kidney, liver and heart transplants are now performed regularly in specialised centres. A working knowledge of basic immune mechanisms is needed to understand the phenomenon of rejection. Both the cell-mediated and humoral arms of the immune response are involved in rejection reactions. The rejection reactions can be classified according to:

1. Whether the response is cell and/or antibody mediated
2. The speed of evolution of the response.

Autoimmune diseases with changed MHC expression	
Disease	**Cells affected**
Graves' disease	Thyroid epithelium
Type 1 diabetes mellitus	Pancreatic B cells
Primary bilary cirrhosis	Bile duct epithelium
Sjögren's syndrome	Salivary ducts

Rheumatoid disease

Definition. Systemic, chronic inflammatory disease. Erroneously called rheumatoid *arthritis*, since blood vessels, kidneys, heart, skin and lungs may also be affected.

Age/sex. Young to middle-aged females. About 1–2% of the adult population are affected worldwide.

Cause. Unknown. However, most patients (~80%) with rheumatoid disease (and particularly joint problems) have circulating autoantibodies (usually IgM) against the Fc region of IgG (rheumatoid factor). It is thought that the disease is initiated by an infectious agent (e.g. virus or bacterium). Rheumatoid disease can be complicated by amyloid deposition (see Ch. 13).

Clinicopathological features:
- Joints — the synovium is initially targeted leading to destruction of cartilage and bone and damage to tendons and ligaments.
- Skin — firm 'rheumatoid nodules' are found in about a quarter of patients, especially on the elbows. These are seen down the microscope as large necrotic areas surrounded by macrophages.
- Blood vessels — vasculitis.
- Lungs, heart, kidney — non-specific inflammation and/or vasculitis.

Clinical course. Variable. There may be a sudden onset of debilitating arthritis or slow, inexorable loss of joint movements. Rarely, patients die from systemic complications (e.g. vasculitis, amyloidosis). Often a variety of powerful anti-inflammatory drug therapies are required to slow disease progression.

Antibody-mediated rejection

A **hyperacute rejection** occurs when a donated organ is placed in a patient who has preformed, circulating antibodies to donor antigens (e.g. multiparous females, multi-transfused patients). The rejection occurs within minutes of the new organ having its blood supply established as antibodies target HLA on the vascular endothelium. Inflammation of vessels, thrombosis and necrosis occur.

Antibody and cell-mediated rejection

Acute cellular rejection

Lymphocytes, plasma cells and blast cells appear within the tissues of the transplanted organ for weeks or months after transplantation and may be related to fluctuations in the level of immunosuppressive drugs. The reaction is caused by the generation of CD8⁺ (cytotoxic) T cells by the recipient which destroy the donor organ. It is possible that dendritic cells within the donor organ are actually responsible for triggering the reaction.

Acute antibody-mediated (vascular) rejection

Recipient antibodies against donor antigens may cause vascular inflammation or intimal proliferation leading to necrosis or obliteration of graft vessels, with tissue loss and scarring. It is common for acute cellular and vascular rejection to co-exist, although one form may dominate.

Cell-mediated rejection

Chronic rejection takes the form of a slow diminution in organ function over time. Characteristically, plasma cells, lymphocytes and eosinophils are seen within the tissue; intimal fibrosis is also prominent. Rejection of grafts can now be prevented, or at least slowed, by a variety of drugs (see the box below).

Prevention and treatment of autograft rejection

1. Reduce graft immunogenicity by:
   - ensuring ABO compatibility
   - 'matching' class I and class II MHC in donor and recipient.

2. Immunosuppression of recipient. The drugs used and their actions are:
   - corticosteroids: cytokine gene transcription blocker (e.g. IL–1)
   - azathiaprine: metabolic toxin stops lymphocyte maturation
   - cyclosporin A: interleukin-2 gene transcription blocker
   - FK506: cytokine gene transcription blocker; less nephrotoxic than cyclosporin A.

   Most drugs act by inhibiting T cell function.

8.4 Immunodeficiency

Immunodeficiency can be classified as congenital (primary) (see the box, right) and acquired (secondary) types. The human immunodeficiency virus (HIV) is responsible for the acquired immunodeficiency syndrome (AIDS) and is now the most important cause of secondary immunodeficiency. The use of immunosuppressive and cytotoxic drugs also gives rise to secondary immunodeficiencies.

AIDS

AIDS is now a massive, world-wide problem. The illness was first recognised in 1981 when a group of homosexual men were noted to have an unusual lung infection (*Pneumocystis carinii pneumonia*). Research into the cause, prevention, mechanisms and treatment of AIDS continues.

Aetiology

AIDS follows, after a varying time interval, infection with a family of retroviruses termed HIV. HIV viruses have distinct genomes but cause similar disease processes.

Pathogenesis

The CD4 molecule of CD4$^+$ T cells acts as a receptor for the HIV allowing it to enter the cell. The virus then uses reverse transcriptase to produce DNA from its own RNA. The viral DNA produced is then inserted into the lymphocyte's chromosomes. The DNA may be transcribed to form more HIV or lie dormant. Tissue macrophages (CD4$^+$) can also be infected. By insertion of viral DNA into the host genome, irreversible and permanent infection of the cell occurs. Direct lysis of CD4$^+$ T cells, the cytopathic effects of integrated viral RNA, DNA and protein, and inhibition of CD4$^+$ T cell maturation as well as autoimmune destruction all contribute to the immunodeficiency. Severe immunosuppression occurs in AIDS patients, leaving them susceptible to a variety of infections and tumours.

Clinical features

Opportunistic infections. These rarely affect immunocompetent individuals but can cause debilitating and fatal illness in patients with AIDS (or immunodeficiency from other causes):

- *Pneumocystis carinii*
- atypical mycobacteria (e.g. *Mycobacterium avium–intracellulare* complex)
- Epstein–Barr virus (EBV)
- herpes simplex virus (HSV)
- cytomegalovirus (CMV).

Tumours. An unusual, probably viral induced, vascular neoplasm called Kaposi's sarcoma may disseminate and kill the patient. Other tumours such as lymphomas (particularly high grade B cell lymphomas, often EBV-related) can also be clinical problems.

Primary immunodeficiencies

Bruton's agammaglobulinaemia
- X linked
- no mature B cells, T cells normal
- recurrent bacterial infections

DiGeorge's syndrome
- mal-development of thymus gland
- no cell mediated response; reduced T cell levels, but normal antibody levels
- recurrent viral, mycobacterial and fungal infections

Severe combined immunodeficiency disease (SCID)
- autosomal recessive and X linked forms
- defect is at the stem cell level; defective T and B cell responses; virtually absent lymphoid tissue
- early death from opportunistic infections

Brain. This is a major site of HIV infection. Most patients develop some form of encephalitis or dementia.

At-risk populations

These include:

- homosexual/bisexual men
- intravenous substance abusers and their contacts
- recipients of blood/blood products, e.g. haemophiliacs prior to introduction of safe blood products.

HIV infection has now spread into the heterosexual population.

Transmission

This is by:

- sexual intercourse (vaginal or anal)
- direct inoculation of the virus through the bloodstream, e.g. needle stick injury
- placenta (mother-to-child).

Natural history

The natural history of AIDS remains to be defined. There is no doubt that patients can remain HIV-positive but AIDS-free for many years. The onset of AIDS, however, usually heralds death within a much shorter time period (depending on response to treatment). The overall prognosis for the disease is still very poor.

Self-assessment: questions

Multiple choice questions

1. The following statements are true:
   a. Asthma is primarily a T cell-mediated immune disease
   b. Skin prick tests are a useful way of predicting immediate hypersensitivity reactions
   c. Rheumatic fever is thought to be immune complex-mediated
   d. Cyclosporin A (immunosuppressive agent) is nephrotoxic
   e. The complement product C3a can cause non-IgE-mediated mast cell degranulation

2. Immune complexes:
   a. Are made up of antigen and antibody
   b. Contain antibody of the IgG class
   c. Are usually insoluble
   d. Combine with complement, which initiates an inflammatory reaction
   e. Are responsible for post-streptococcal glomerulonephritis

Case history

A 26-year-old rhesus-negative woman with a 20-week pregnancy was admitted to an obstetric observation unit. She had not felt the baby move for 3 days. An ultrasound scan confirmed the baby was dead and a stillborn baby was born. At post-mortem, the baby was swollen and had massive pleural effusions and ascites. A high level of anti-D antibodies was detected in the mother's blood. The father had a blood test which showed him to be O rhesus-positive (probably DD). The woman had had three previous pregnancies by the same man. The first baby was completely normal.

1. What was the underlying immunological process which led to the death of the baby?
2. Why were there no problems with the first baby?
3. Give two other examples of this type of hypersensitivity reaction.

Short notes

Write short notes on the following:

1. AIDS
2. Autoimmune disease
3. Type 1 hypersensitivity reactions (asthma)
4. Haemolytic disease of the newborn
5. Important cells in transplant rejection reactions.

Self-assessment: answers

Multiple choice answers

1. a. **False.** Asthma is a disease caused by an immediate hypersensitivity reaction, mediated by IgE. The intense bronchoconstriction which causes the breathlessness and wheezing results from the action of smooth muscle contractors released by the degranulation of mast cells.

   b. **True.** If a small amount of allergen such as house dust or pollen is injected into the skin in a person already sensitised to the substance, i.e. who already has IgE antibodies against the substance, an immediate wheal and flare reaction will occur. This clinical test is a useful way of predicting hypersensitivity reactions and also of determining which antigens are likely to trigger them.

   c. **False.** Rheumatic fever can be considered an immune-mediated disease triggered by a bacterial infection. The disease often affects children and usually follows a few weeks after a group A streptococcal sore throat. It is believed that, during the course of the immune response to the streptococcus, either antibodies are produced which cross-react with the body's own tissues or the infection 'triggers' an autoimmune disease. In either case, there follows an acute febrile illness which may involve the joints, heart and brain.

   d. **True.** By mechanisms which are as yet uncertain, cyclosporin A damages the kidney. Careful monitoring of the blood levels of the drug and function of the kidneys is required.

   e. **True.** There are a variety of substances which cause degranulation of mast cells independent of IgE. These include the complement components C3a and C5a (the anaphylatoxins), drugs such as morphine and physical stimuli such as extreme heat and cold.

2. a. **True.** Classical experiments in the 1960s and 1970s showed that if rabbits are injected with bovine serum albumin (BSA), they quickly produce anti-BSA antibodies, and immune complexes of BSA–anti-BSA form. These initially circulate in the bloodstream and are then deposited in tissues (e.g. glomerulus).

   b. **True.** IgG is nearly always the antibody involved in complex formation.

   c. **False.** Small soluble complexes are the ones which deposit in blood vessel walls and cause damage. Large insoluble complexes are easily phagocytosed and removed by tissue macrophages.

   d. **True.** Tissue damage occurs following the classical pathway of complement activation.

   e. **True.** Soluble immune complexes composed of IgG and streptococcal antigen deposit in the glomerular capillary loops and initiate a complement-mediated inflammatory reaction. Alternatively, if some streptococcal antigens are positively charged they may 'stick' in the negatively charged matrix of the glomerulus and in situ immune complex formation occurs. There is damage to the glomerular basement membrane and neutrophils and macrophages are recruited to the site. Immune complexes can be visualised in tissue sections of the glomerulus by immunofluorescent or immunohistochemical techniques (see Chapter 2).

Case history answer

1 & 2. This baby died of haemolytic disease of the newborn (HDN), in this case caused by rhesus incompatibility. If a fetus inherits paternal red cell rhesus antigens that are foreign to the mother's immune system, reaction to these antigens may occur. At the time of birth, leakage of the baby's red cells into the maternal circulation occurs. This leads to an immune response by, and sensitisation of, the mother. Although there will be no effect on the first baby, who will be a week or two old by this time, subsequent rhesus-positive fetuses will be at risk. If fetal blood crosses into the mother's circulation during a subsequent pregnancy, maternal IgG anti-D antibodies will quickly be produced. IgG antibodies can cross the placenta and fix to the antigen on fetal red cells, causing them to be rapidly destroyed (haemolysed). In severe cases, there is hypoxic injury to the heart and liver. Liver failure results in reduced production of albumin with consequent reduced oncotic pressure and thus oedema (ascites and pleural effusions lead to the swollen appearance of the baby). The destruction of red cells produces high levels of circulating unconjugated bilirubin, which can deposit in and damage the brain, causing fits and death if untreated.

   As a reaction to the loss of red cells, a phenomenon known as extramedullary haemopoiesis (EMH) occurs. Bone marrow elements producing red cells, white cells and platelets are present in sites other than the medullary cavities of bones. In severe HDN, there are red cell precursors in the liver, spleen, skin and many other organs, in an attempt to maintain red cell numbers and circulating and tissue oxygen levels. Widespread EMH is normally only seen in the first and second trimesters when the fetus cannot fully depend on bone marrow precursors for blood formation. Sites of EMH are mainly the liver, spleen and yolk sac. Some EMH is seen in full-term infants, but the bone marrow takes over soon after birth.

Not all cases of HDN are caused by rhesus incompatibility. In fact, ABO incompatibility is more common but very rarely causes clinical problems, partly because the antibodies are IgM and cannot cross the placenta.

The routine administration of anti-D immunoglobulin to women soon after birth means that rhesus incompatibility is now a rare clinical problem.

3. Rhesus incompatibility is an example of a type 2 hypersensitivity reaction. Other examples include incompatible blood transfusion reaction (blood group ABO antigens) and some autoimmune haemolytic anaemias.

Short notes answers

1. Cover HIV infection, the pathogenesis and natural history of the disease, including the method of transmission and the at-risk population. Describe the clinical features.

2. In autommine disease antibodies are formed against the patient's own tissues; it can affect one particular cell type, one organ system or many organs (multi-system). These reactions do not normally occur: tolerance. Autoimmune disease is associated with changes in MHC expression, both increased expression and expression on cells that would normally be negative for that class of MHC

molecule. Use SLE and rheumatoid disease as examples.

3. Discuss the various aspects of type 1 hypersensitivity:

- IgE-mediated
- immediate
- degranulation of mast cells
- smooth muscle contractions
- role of histamine.

Use asthma, hay fever and generalised anaphylaxis as examples.

4. Haemolytic disease of the newborn occurs in a rhesus-positive fetus carried by a rhesus-negative mother; it affects babies subsequent to the first pregnancy, which is usually normal. Maternal antibodies are produced as a result of leakage of fetal cells into the maternal circulation: anti-D antibodies. In subsequent pregnancies, these antibodies cause haemolysis of fetal cells. This can be prevented by injecting the mother with IgG rhesus antibody immediately after each delivery to 'mop up' any fetal cells and prevent her producing natural antibody.

5. Cells involved in transplant rejection reactions include:

- CD8⁺ cytotoxic T cells
- donor dendritic cells
- vascular endothelial cells.

Therapies (immunosuppressive drugs) are aimed at paralysing/destroying the T cell immune reaction.

Inflammation

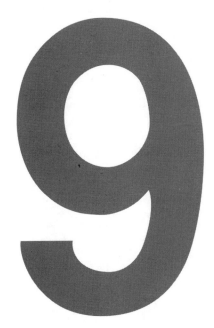

Chapter overview

Inflammatory processes are part of the body's natural defences. The beneficial effects of localising the damage/infection can be accompanied by deleterious tissue damage.

9.1 Cellular processes of inflammation

Inflammation is the most important of the body's defence mechanisms. Inflammation is the local response to injury in living, vascularised tissues. Its purpose is to localise and eliminate the injurious agent and then to restore the tissue to normal structure and function. However, inflammation may be seen as a process like a two-edged sword. On the one hand, it has beneficial effects by localising and 'walling off' an infection; on the other, it may be detrimental to the host and cause extensive tissue damage. Inflamed tissues are named with the suffix 'itis'; thus appendicitis is inflammation of the appendix and hepatitis is inflammation of the liver.

Causes of inflammation:

- microbial infections: bacteria, viruses, fungi
- hypersensitivity reactions: types I–IV
- physical agents: burns, UV light, radiation
- chemicals: acids, alkalis, oxidising agents
- tissue necrosis: ischaemia.

Symptoms and signs of inflammation:

- redness from dilatation of blood vessels
- pain from oedema, histamine release
- heat/fever from vasodilatation, release of pyrogens
- swelling from oedema
- loss of function from pain and swelling.

Cells of the inflammatory response

Neutrophil polymorphs
Neutrophils are the first cells to appear at the site of acute inflammation. Their function is to degrade cell debris and to ingest and kill microbes (phagocytosis). Neutrophils originate in the bone marrow and have a short tissue life span of only 3–4 days. They contain bactericidal intracellular enzymes in lysosomes:

- myeloperoxidase
- lysozyme
- acid hydrolase.

The lysosomes fuse with the vacuole containing the ingested material, releasing the enzymes which can destroy the contents.

Eosinophils
These phagocytic cells originate in the bone marrow and have striking red/pink intracytoplasmic granules when visualised using a haematoxylin and eosin stain. They are associated with type I hypersensitivity responses and produce substances which 'damp down' allergic inflammatory reactions. Thus, they produce histaminase, aryl sulphatase and phospholipase, which degrade anaphylactic chemical mediators, particularly those produced by mast cells.

Basophils and mast cells
Mast cells are usually seen in tissues in type I hypersensitivity reactions mediated by IgE. Mast cells have IgE Fc receptors on their cell membranes. Basophils and mast cells both have cytoplasmic granules which contain heparin and histamine and enzymes such as tryptase and acid hydrolase. Binding of IgE to the Fc receptors leads to degranulation and release of the granule contents into the tissues.

Monocytes and macrophages
Macrophages are the major scavenger cells of the body. They are derived from blood monocytes and are attracted to sites of inflammation by chemotactic factors, appearing 12–24 hours later than neutrophils. Macrophages are long-lived phagocytic cells and contain powerful intracellular enzymes and chemicals (lysozyme and hydrogen peroxide) which degrade particulate matter including dead neutrophils and microorganisms. They orchestrate many of the cellular, vascular and reparative responses of inflammation by releasing chemotactic factors such as neutrophil chemotactic factor, coagulation factors (factor VIII), cytokines (tumour necrosis factor) and growth factors (PDGF and transforming growth factor beta (TGF-β)).

Lymphocytes and plasma cells
These are the principal cells of many of the specific immune responses but are also seen in general inflammatory reactions.

Control of recruitment of inflammatory cells to sites of inflammation

Until recently, the cellular processes controlling the sticking of neutrophils and monocytes to the endothelium at sites of inflammation were poorly understood. It is now known that interactions can occur between different cells and between cells and connective tissue. These interactions, however brief, involve cell adhesion molecules (CAMs). These link to one another in a similar manner to a lock and key. Cell adhesion molecules are involved in a wide variety of cellular processes, such as inflammation, cell locomotion, tumour spread and immune mechanisms. Details of the names, classes and functions of CAMs are probably unnecessary at undergraduate level, but the principles of the mechanisms of action are important to understand.

In inflammation, vascular endothelial cells can display adhesion molecules which will bind to neutrophils and monocytes. Some of the CAMs are already present within the endothelial cell and are redistributed to the surface, others are newly produced. Many of the chemical mediators of inflammation trigger endothelial cells to produce CAMs. In addition, neutrophils and monocytes also have surface adhesion molecules (integrins). Some integrins are always present on the cell surface, but will only become 'sticky' when the cell enters a site of inflammation, causing strong binding with its ligand on the endothelial surface.

9.2 Types of inflammation

Acute inflammation

Acute inflammation is defined as the early inflammatory response to an injurious agent, which is characterised by the presence of neutrophil polymorphs and later macrophages. Acute inflammation usually lasts for a few hours or days and then resolves, leaving little or no permanent tissue damage.

The early acute inflammatory response is characterised by the presence of oedema fluid, fibrin and neutrophil polymorphs in the extracellular spaces of the injured tissue (Fig. 22). This is caused by:

- arteriolar dilatation and opening up of capillary channels
- increased vascular permeability (exudate formation)
- emigration of neutrophils from vessels.

Vasodilatation
This occurs rapidly in the early inflammatory response and leads to increased blood flow into the damaged

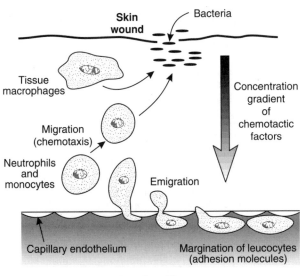

Fig. 22
Acute inflammation.

tissue. Dilatation may last from 15 minutes to several hours, depending on the severity of the injury.

Increased vascular permeability
Venules and capillaries are lined by a continuous layer of endothelium which keeps blood cells and large proteins within the vessel. In acute inflammation, the intravascular hydrostatic pressure increases and gaps appear between endothelial cells, allowing fluid and proteins (exudate) to leak into the extracellular tissues. Within the dilated vascular beds, blood flow will slow dramatically as protein-rich fluid is lost into tissues and blood cells mass within the vessels.

Emigration of neutrophils
The protein and cell-rich exudate is the hallmark of inflammation and is composed of plasma proteins (mainly fibrin) mixed with neutrophils in the extracellular space. The following stages occur in this process:

1. Margination of neutrophils: reduced blood flow and increased viscosity in the dilated capillaries cause neutrophils to flow close to the vessel wall in the plasmatic zone and not centrally (axial flow).
2. Pavementing of neutrophils: neutrophils adhere to the endothelium (adhesion molecules).
3. Emigration of neutrophils: neutrophils use active amoeboid movement to pass through endothelial gaps. They are attracted by high concentrations of chemotactic bacterial products and complement proteins (C5a) and cytokines (e.g. interleukins) outside the vessel. The neutrophils 'sense' these agents by cell surface receptors.
4. A process called diapedesis also occurs. This is the term usually given to the passive leakage of red blood cells through the leaky vessel wall.

Tissue events
Once the neutrophils and monocytes have left the vascular compartment and travelled by chemotaxis-stimulated movement to the site of tissue injury, their main role in inflammation becomes evident. Neutrophils and macrophages can recognise, engulf, internalise and enzymatically destroy microorganisms or other foreign materials, as well as host cells (Fig. 23).

Chemical mediators
These have an important role in orchestrating the inflammatory response. They are widely distributed throughout the body in an inactive form and are released, synthesised or activated locally at the site of inflammation (Table 13). Inactivation occurs rapidly after release, which is important for the control and localisation of inflammation.

Outcomes of acute inflammation
Resolution. Acute inflammation usually disappears after a few days and the tissue returns to normal. Fluid and degraded proteins are drained by the lymphatic

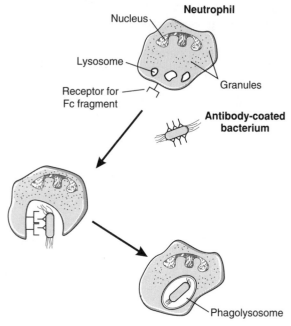

Neutrophil

Nucleus

Lysosome

Receptor for
Fc fragment

Granules

**Antibody-coated
bacterium**

Phagolysosome

Fig. 23
Phagocytosis. Phagocytic cells ingest cell debris and microbes,
which are digested in vacuoles by lysosomal enzymes.

channels and the exudate, cell debris and fibrin are
removed by neutrophils and monocytes. To prevent further acute inflammation occurring, the inflammatory
cells are finally removed by apoptosis.

Progression to chronic inflammation. As a result of
persistent inflammatory stimuli the inflammatory
process can move into a chronic phase.

Chronic inflammation

Chronic inflammation is an inflammatory response
characterised by the presence of lymphocytes, plasma
cells and macrophages. It may arise from unresolved
acute inflammation or de novo. Chronic inflammation
may go on for months or even years and will nearly
always leave behind areas of permanent tissue damage.

Clinically, chronic inflammation may occur as a
result of:

- a persistent inflammatory stimulus, e.g. foreign
body, including surgical sutures
- recurrent bouts of acute inflammation, e.g. episodes
of gallbladder inflammation (cholecystitis) caused
by gall stones
- low-grade inflammation caused by infection (e.g.
tuberculosis) or by autoimmune reactions (e.g.
rheumatoid arthritis).

Chronic inflammation may persist for weeks,
months or years and is recognised by:

- infiltration by macrophages, lymphocytes and
plasma cells, i.e. chronic inflammatory cells, with
only a scanty population of neutrophils
- tissue destruction with proliferation of fibroblasts
and small blood vessels (granulation tissue) and
production of collagen (scar) tissue.

Macrophages play a key role in chronic inflammation, as they do in the latter stages of acute inflammation. The preferential accumulation of macrophages in
chronic inflammation is at least partly a result of the
profile of adhesion molecules displayed by the endothelium in the damaged area. Macrophages will also proliferate locally and, being long-lived, become the
dominant cell population.

Macrophages can produce a range of substances.
Particularly important in chronic inflammation are the
'pro-fibrosis' molecules, such as growth factors (particularly transforming growth factor beta) and certain
cytokines. The conversion of granulation tissue into
scar tissue is dealt with in Chapter 10.

Table 13 Chemical mediators involved in inflammation

Mediator	Source	Function
Histamine and serotonin	Mast cells and basophils, platelets	Vasodilatation and early increase in vascular permeability
Lysosomal compounds (acid hydrolases/ tissue proteases)	Neutrophils, macrophages	Increase vascular permeability, activate complement, increase damage
Prostaglandins (PGs) and PG-like substances	Arachidonic acid derived from cell membrane phospholipid	PGE_2 and PGI_2 from endothelium cause vasodilatation, thromboxane A_2 from platelets causes vasoconstriction
Nitric oxide	Vascular endothelium macrophages	Vasodilatation, toxic to bacteria
Platelet activating factor (PAF)	Most white cells, vascular endothelium	Increases vascular permeability, increases adhesion of white cells to endothelium and induces platelet aggregation
Leukotrienes	Neutrophils	Neutrophil chemotaxis, vasoconstriction, increased vascular permeability
Cytokines	Lymphocytes, macrophages	IL-1, TNF and IL-8 are involved in endothelial cell activation, chemotaxis and fever

Granulomatous inflammation

This is a special type of chronic inflammation in which macrophages accumulate and undergo special morphological and functional changes (Fig. 24). Macrophages may transform into epithelioid macrophages or fuse to form giant cells. Giant cells are large cells with between 10–100 nuclei (multinucleated cells). An aggregate of epithelioid cells, often containing giant cells, is called a granuloma. Epithelioid macrophages have a secretory morphology, i.e. abundant ribosomes and endoplasmic reticulum and only limited phagocytic capabilities.

Macrophages can be stimulated to form granulomas by:

- indigestible organisms, e.g. mycobacteria (TB and leprosy)
- foreign material, e.g. silica, carbon (tattoos), talc, suture material
- unknown mechanisms, e.g. in rheumatoid arthritis, sarcoidosis.

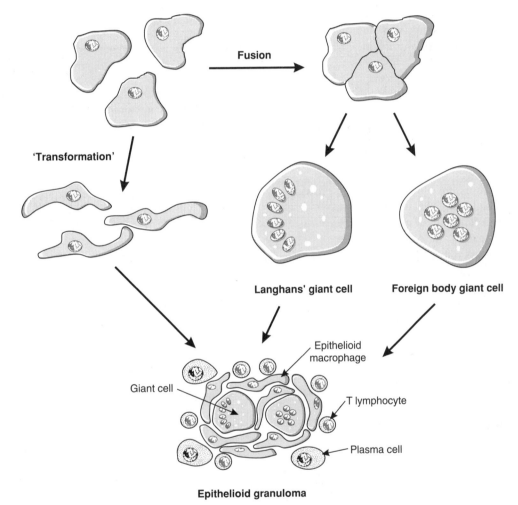

Fig. 24
Giant cells and the granuloma.

Self-assessment: questions

Multiple choice questions

1. During the acute inflammatory response:
   a. Histamine causes vasodilatation
   b. The exuded fibrin is formed by local fibroblasts
   c. Margination of monocytes is an early event
   d. Red cell diapedesis is a passive phenomenon
   e. Complement components may act as chemo-attractants

2. The following are correctly paired:
   a. Granulomatous inflammation — *Mycobacterium tuberculosis*
   b. Plasma cells — phagocytosis
   c. Pus — collection of neutrophils
   d. Eosinophils — parasitic infection
   e. Langerhans' giant cells — *Mycobacterium tuberculosis*

3. The following statements are correct:
   a. An inflammatory exudate is rich in protein
   b. Giant cells result from fusion of lymphocytes
   c. Acute inflammation usually progresses to chronic inflammation
   d. An abscess is a collection of walled-off pus
   e. Macrophages are derived from blood monocytes

Case histories

Case history 1

> A 10-year-old girl is admitted to hospital with a 3-day history of right iliac fossa pain, associated with a fever. Examination reveals severe abdominal tenderness. Appendicectomy is performed. At operation, the tip of the appendix is swollen and covered in a purulent exudate.

1. What are the likely histological features of the tip of the appendix?
2. Why might the girl have had a high temperature?
3. What are the likely outcomes of acute appendicitis?

Case history 2

> A 63-year-old man has part of his large bowel removed through an abdominal incision. Five days after operation, the wound is red, hot and painful and pus is seen coming out from one end.

1. What is likely to have happened?

> After appropriate treatment, the wound heals and a scar forms. However, a small, firm area within the scar causes the man some discomfort and this is removed about 2 years after his original operation. The histology report states 'a foreign body giant cell reaction to suture (stitch) material seen'.

2. What is a foreign body giant cell reaction?
3. What other types of giant cell are there?

Short notes

Write short notes on the following:

1. The cells of the inflammatory reaction
2. Chemotaxis
3. Advantages and disadvantages of inflammation.

Viva questions

1. What is chronic inflammation?
2. What is the role of neutrophils/macrophages?
3. Discuss the role of cell mediators.

Self-assessment: answers

Multiple choice answers

1. a. **True.** Histamine is a vasoactive amine secreted by mast cells. It acts via receptors on post-capillary venules during the early phase of acute inflammation to increase permeability of the vessel.

   b. **False.** This is a common examiner's trick. Fibroblasts secrete procollagen, which is converted to collagen outside the cell. In fact *no* cells produce fibrin; fibrin is derived from fibrinogen, a hepatocyte-derived clotting factor.

   c. **False.** Margination of cells is an early event in acute inflammation, but it is the neutrophil polymorph that is recruited initially and not the monocyte.

   d. **True.** Whereas the process of neutrophil emigration is an active, 'purposeful' phenomenon, red cells leave the vessel as a result of the combined effects of raised intravascular hydrostatic pressure and vascular leakiness.

   e. **True.** Chemotaxis is the unidirectional, purposeful flow of neutrophils or macrophages towards a chemo-attractant. The cells often have receptors for the coated molecule on their surfaces. Components of the complement pathway such as C5a can attract inflammatory cells such as neutrophils into the inflamed area.

2. a. **True.** Tuberculosis is a classical example of a chronic granulomatous inflammatory disease. In the typical example of TB, the granuloma shows central caseous necrosis (see Ch. 4).

   b. **False.** Phagocytosis is the process by which neutrophils and macrophages engulf and then dispose of particulate material. Plasma cells have no such ability; their function is to produce antibody.

   c. **True.** Pus is a collection of viable and dead or dying neutrophils, often admixed with the non-viable tissue in which the acute inflammatory reaction has occurred. Thus, pus formation is another consequence of acute inflammation.

   d. **True.** Eosinophils are often the dominant inflammatory cells involved in parasitic infections. It is thought that eosinophil products make the microenvironment around the parasites unsuitable for their continuing survival.

   e. **False.** This is a common misconception. The giant cells in a TB granuloma are known as Langhans' giant cells not Langerhan's cells, which are dendritic antigen-presenting cells in the epidermis.

3. a. **True.** The inflammatory exudate results from the process of increased vascular permeability where plasma proteins and inflammatory cells move out into the injured tissues. The exudate is, therefore, rich in fibrinogen, which then becomes converted to a fibrin meshwork. This inhibits the movement of organisms and gives phagocytes a supporting structure. In contrast, a transudate is composed of oedema fluid which leaks out of capillaries as a result of an increase in hydrostatic pressure. Transudates are low in protein.

   b. **False.** Giant cells are usually formed by the fusion of macrophages in response to immune stimuli or foreign bodies. In other circumstances, giant cells may form in malignant tumours by abnormal mitotic division of epithelial or mesenchymal cells. These are called tumour giant cells.

   c. **False.** Acute inflammation usually resolves, with restoration of normal structure and function. Sometimes, it will progress to chronic inflammation. This depends on a variety of factors, such as the presence of a persistent injurious stimulus, particularly a pathogenic organism.

   d. **True.** Infection with pyogenic organisms such as *Staphylococcus aureus* causes suppurative inflammation. Pus may form diffusely in tissue planes, or collect in discrete foci, which may become walled-off by fibrin, granulation tissue and eventually fibrous scarring. An abscess wall effectively isolates the infected locus, preventing the body's inflammatory cells from reaching it and also preventing antibiotics from being effective. This is why surgical intervention to drain the abscess is the most effective treatment.

   e. **True.** Blood monocytes migrate through the walls of venules to inflamed tissue. Once in the tissue they are known as macrophages and have an important phagocytic function. Some tissues and organs in the body contain a population of 'resident' macrophages which originally derived from the bone marrow. Examples of these include alveolar macrophages, Kupffer cells of the liver and Langerhans' cells of the skin.

Case history answers

Case history 1

1. Acute appendicitis is one of the most common causes of abdominal pain encountered clinically, and appendicectomy is one of the most frequent emergency operations. To the naked eye, an appendix showing established acute inflammation will have a stringy, greenish exudate on the surface

and the wall will be pale, firm and swollen. Debris or faecal material (a faecalith) may be found in the lumen. Microscopically, the outer surface may be coated with pus and fibrin, the wall will be oedematous and neutrophils will be seen in appendiceal glands and muscle. Small aggregates of neutrophils may form (micro-abscesses). The lumen may contain purulent fluid and debris.

2. A high temperature (fever, pyrexia) and a general feeling of being unwell (malaise) often accompany acute inflammation, particularly fulminant cases. There is no doubt that some bacterial products (exogenous pyrogens, e.g. endotoxin) stimulate white cells to produce substances (endogenous pyrogens, e.g. interleukin-1, interleukin-6 and tumour necrosis factor) which act at the level of the hypothalamus to increase body temperature. The systemic effects of inflammation (weight loss, altered liver function) are probably all mediated by cytokines.

3. Despite being such a common surgical condition, little is known about the natural history of acute appendicitis. It is possible that resolution occurs in mild early cases; in others, recurrent inflammation can lead to a small, scarred appendix. The most serious outcome can be predicted from a knowledge of basic pathological processes. The appendiceal wall may soften, become necrotic and rupture occurs. Acute inflammation of the peritoneum (peritonitis) follows and septicaemia (multiplying bacteria in the bloodstream) will ensue. The latter will be fatal without treatment. Even in the 1990s, a small number of patients die from this. Other outcomes include the acute inflammatory process spreading to adjacent structures and an abscess or appendiceal mass forming.

Case history 2

1. Again, this is a common clinical situation and shows how a knowledge of basic pathological processes is important in clinical medicine. Post-operative wound infections, particularly after large abdominal operations, are rare but require prompt action. The man's wound site exhibits some of the cardinal signs of acute inflammation. In addition, pus is seen issuing from the wound. Swabs of the pus and wound edges should be taken for identification of the bacteria causing the inflammatory process; they may originate from bowel or skin flora.

2. Foreign material may be retained within the body, particularly inert material that cannot be degraded by phagocytic cells, such as insoluble suture material or talc. This evokes a granulomatous response. Within the granuloma, foreign body giant cells are often seen. These have large numbers of nuclei scattered throughout the cytoplasm. In contrast, Langhans' giant cells, seen in TB, have a horse shoe arrangement of nuclei around the periphery of the cell (see Fig. 24).

3. Giant cells are disproportionately large cells that have numerous nuclei (multinucleate giant cells). The classical multinucleate giant cells are Langhans' (TB, sarcoid), foreign body (sutures, talc) (Fig. 24) and Touton. Touton giant cells are seen in lipid-containing lesions such as xanthelasma and areas of fat necrosis. They have a central, ring-like arrangement of nuclei and peripheral fat droplets in their cytoplasm. Not all large, multinucleated cells are giant cells in a pathological sense. Examples include bone-resorbing osteoclasts and platelet-producing megakaryocytes.

Short notes answers

1. First of all, define the inflammatory reaction and then list the main cellular components of the inflammatory reaction and state their origin, function and sequence of appearance. For example, neutrophils are derived from myeloid stem cells in the bone marrow and are present in circulating blood. They are the first cells to arrive at the site of acute inflammation and exit from venules by a process known as emigration. They produce enzymes and are phagocytic so that they have an important function in removing dead cells and microorganisms. Use a diagram to illustrate this (e.g. Fig. 22).

2. Chemotaxis is a process whereby the leucocyte is attracted along a concentration gradient of a chemotactic factor. Give examples of these, such as bacterial fragments, complement factor C5a, leukotrienes and cytokines, e.g. interleukin-8.

3. Define inflammation, how it occurs, why and what components are involved.

   Advantages:

   - allows damaged tissue to be restored to normal or repaired
   - allows foreign tissue and organisms to be diluted by oedema fluid and removed by cells
   - localises the infection.

   Disadvantages:

   - painful
   - may not result in perfect healing and thus lead to scarring
   - may lead to destruction of adjacent innocent bystander cells tissues.

Viva answers

1. Chronic inflammation may arise de novo or be a result of chronic irritation or non-resolving acute inflammation. It is characterised by its high content of macrophages and lymphocytes and plasma cells.

It may contain granulomas. For example, TB is a chronic granulomatous condition that arises de novo; chronic cholecystitis is caused by gall stones irritating the gallbladder mucosa. Chronic inflammation usually leads to fibrosis and scarring.

2. Neutrophils and macrophages leave the vascular compartment and travel by chemotaxis-stimulated movement to the site of tissue injury. Their main role in inflammation is to recognise, engulf, internalise and destroy microorganisms or other foreign materials, as well as host cells (See Fig. 23).

3. Cell mediators are groups of molecules known as cytokines or lymphokines. They send signals between cells and orchestrate the inflammatory, immune and repair processes. Examples include interleukins and interferons.

Healing and repair

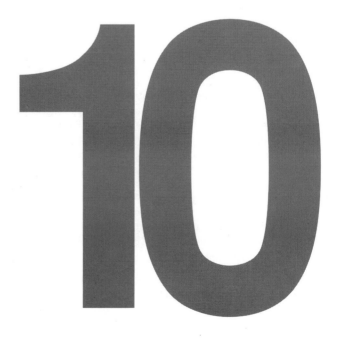

Chapter overview

Healing is the replacement of dead or injured tissue by healthy tissue; this is accomplished by regeneration, when the damage is mild and labile cells are involved, and by repair, which includes the formation of granulation tissue and then a scar. Repair occurs with extensive tissue injury or in permanent cell populations.

10.1 Healing

Healing, regeneration and repair are terms which are often used synonymously. This is incorrect and can be confusing. Healing is a general term for the processes involved in the replacement of dead and injured tissue by healthy tissue. Regeneration and repair are the two processes whereby this is accomplished. Regeneration is the replacement of dead cells by an exactly similar living cell population, whereas repair involves the production of scar tissue to replace dead cells. Repair will always occur when the normal connective tissue matrix around cells is destroyed.

When does healing occur?

Healing occurs in all damaged tissues. It begins early in the inflammatory reaction, when macrophages phagocytose debris and clear the way for healing to occur. If the injury is mild then healing takes place by regeneration and replacement of injured tissue with cells of the same type, leaving no trace of damage. This is more likely to occur in labile or stable cell populations. In more severe or chronic types of injury, or in permanent cell populations, healing takes place by fibrosis (scarring, repair). This results in loss of specialised cells and hence loss of function, although structural integrity is preserved.

Examples of when healing occurs are:

- skin wounds
- bone fractures
- inflammatory reactions
- myocardial infarction.

The healing of skin wounds has been extensively studied and much of our understanding of the healing process comes from observation of surgical skin wounds. The central pathological process in healing is the formation of granulation tissue.

What is granulation tissue?

This bright pink, granular tissue is characteristically seen in the base of a skin wound and denotes the healing process. Granulation tissue is composed of:

- small blood vessels (capillary sized channels)
- proliferating (myo)fibroblasts.

New blood vessels develop from budding of pre-existing capillaries (neovascularisation) in the surrounding undamaged tissues. Initially solid, they soon open into capillary loops at the edges of the lesion accompanied by new lymphatic channels. Fibroblasts migrate to the area, transforming into myofibroblasts which contain bundles of muscle-like filaments. The fibroblasts produce collagen and contract to reduce the wound size. Although initially granulation tissue is composed of a watery collection of inflammatory cells (neutrophils, macrophages) and proliferating vascular channels and fibroblasts, in the course of a few weeks it becomes an acellular scar, rich in collagen. The capillary channels die away and the (myo)fibroblasts become inactive. Eventually an avascular fibrous scar is formed (organisation).

How is granulation tissue formation controlled?

Growth factors and cytokines orchestrate the cellular events in healing. Regeneration of the epidermis is mediated by epidermal growth factor (EGF), produced by epidermal cells around the damaged area. Neovascularisation is triggered by fibroblast growth factor (FGF) and endothelial growth factors which are produced by macrophages. Fibroblast activity is mediated by FGF and transforming growth factor beta (TGF-β), again derived from macrophages, and platelet-derived growth factor (PDGF) from platelets in the clot or scab in the wound.

Examples of types of tissue healing

Skin wound healing

A simple incised surgical wound will heal by 'primary intention'. This means that the clean edges of a wound once apposed will heal quickly with minimal granulation tissue formation and thus minimal scarring (Fig. 25A). There are several stages:

1. Blood escapes from damaged vessels and fills the gap.
2. Fibrin clot binds the edges together loosely and dries on the surface, forming a scab.
3. An acute inflammatory reaction develops around the wound in 24 hours and the exudate adds more fibrin, polymorphs and macrophages to the wound. These produce lytic enzymes which start to digest any clot and remove any debris from the wound site.
4. Epithelial cells start to regenerate and bridge the gap within 48 hours.
5. Fibrin in the wound provides stability so that blood vessels can regrow and a small amount of granulation tissue may form. The final scar will be very inconspicuous.

Healing by secondary intention

If the wound is large and gaping, infected or there is substantial tissue loss, e.g. a large burn or ulcer, then

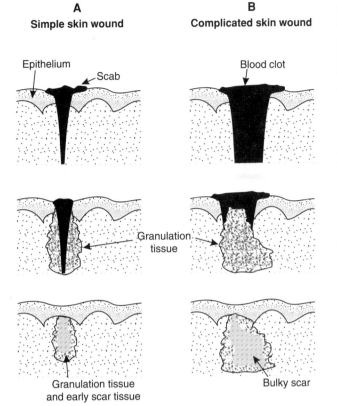

A
Simple skin wound

B
Complicated skin wound

Fig. 25
Wound healing. A. Healing by primary intention. B. Healing by secondary intention.

healing by secondary intention takes place (Fig. 25B). More granulation tissue forms at the base of the wound and fills it up. Epithelial cells can then regenerate over this 'bridge'. Fibroblasts migrate into the wound and, by about day 4, begin producing type III collagen, stimulated by FGF, TGF-β and PDGF. Type III collagen has a low tensile strength but binds the edges of the wound together. Type III collagen is gradually converted to type I collagen, which is stronger and with time aligns itself along lines of stress.

Collagen is degraded by a family of enzymes known as metalloproteinases (e.g. collagenase and elastase), which are produced by cells such as macrophages and fibroblasts. These enzymes are quickly inhibited by another set of enzymes, produced by most connective tissue cells (tissue inhibitors of metalloproteinases).

Bone fracture healing

When a bone breaks, the two ends must be apposed for optimum healing to occur. Local haemorrhage (haematoma) allows modified granulation tissue to grow around the fracture site. This modified granulation tissue consists of proliferating periosteum-derived cells which differentiate into chondroblasts, osteoblasts and fibroblasts (callus). New bone can then be laid down and remodelled and ultimately perfect bony union of the bone ends will occur.

Gastrointestinal tract

Damage to the mucosa of the gastrointestinal tract rapidly heals by epithelial regeneration. If injury

involves the submucosa or deeper muscle layers, then healing occurs by granulation tissue formation and scarring, with re-epithelialisation at the surface. A break in the epithelial surface is known as an erosion. An ulcer is the term given to a defect of the bowel lining which extends deeper into the wall.

Factors affecting wound healing

A variety of factors will adversely affect healing and repair.

Local factors

Tissue apposition. The edges of a wound or a broken bone need to be closely aligned for effective healing to occur.

Infection. An infected wound or tissue will take longer to heal (if at all).

Dead tissue. This must be removed surgically (debridement) or naturally by phagocytosis (macrophages, neutrophils) before healing can be completed.

Blood supply. Ischaemic tissues do not heal properly.

General factors

Dietary. An adequate diet is important to ensure regeneration processes can occur.

Scurvy. Vitamin C deficiency leads to inadequate collagen formation and poor healing.

Starvation/malnutrition. Lack of dietary proteins inhibits wound healing.

Therapy. Many modern therapeutic treatments may adversely affect a particular stage of the healing process.

Steroids. Steroids inhibit the growth of new blood vessels and many macrophage functions. This occurs with long-term steroid therapy and in Cushing's syndrome, where excessive amounts of endogenous steroid are produced.

Immunosuppressive drugs. These will prevent the natural immune response involved in healing.

Anti-cancer drugs. Many anti-cancer drugs inhibit stages in the cell cycle or kill cells involved in active proliferation.

Radiotherapy. Radiotherapy also destroys cells actively dividing.

General cardiovascular status. Poor cardiac function with generalised, severe atherosclerosis leads to an inadequate blood supply to wounded tissues, especially in the distal lower limb.

Systemic disease. Many systemic diseases have secondary effects that adversely affect healing and repair, e.g. diabetes mellitus, haematological diseases and immunosuppression.

10.2 Scarring

Scarring is not only unsightly, it may have serious consequences. Scar tissue tends to contract with time and will not function in the same way as the surrounding tissue. Examples of this include:

- skin contractures following severe burns
- fibrous narrowing (stricture formation) of the duodenum following healing of a peptic ulcer
- ventricular dilatation (aneurysm formation) following myocardial infarction and scarring.

Self-assessment: questions

Multiple choice questions

1. The essential components of granulation tissue are:
   a. Epithelioid macrophages and giant cells
   b. Mast cells
   c. Capillary buds
   d. Fibroblasts
   e. Lymphocytes

2. A deficiency of the following is known to impair wound healing:
   a. Vitamin C
   b. Lead
   c. Vitamin B_{12}
   d. Zinc
   e. Corticosteroids

3. The following are correctly paired:
   a. Labile cells — scarring
   b. Regeneration — permanent cells
   c. Normal epithelium — contact inhibition
   d. Bowel obstruction — stricture
   e. Wound haematoma — organisation

Case histories

Case history 1

A 37-year-old fireman suffers small areas of full thickness burns to the skin of his hands, face and neck during the course of his duties.

1. What is a full thickness skin burn and how might it heal?

Six months after this episode, he develops pain in his neck at the site of the burn scar. The scar and skin around it appear twisted and distorted.

2. Describe the maturation of granulation tissue into scar tissue. What is the complication of the scarring process seen in the fireman called? What other abnormalities of the granulation tissue–scar tissue process can occur?

Case history 2

An 89-year-old diabetic woman in poor general health falls in the street and suffers a compound fracture of her lower right forearm.

1. What local and systemic factors may be important in the healing of the fracture in this patient?

Despite appropriate management of the fracture, the woman finds it difficult to use her arm and becomes bed-ridden. Ten days after her operation, she is found dead in bed.

2. What is the likely cause of death?

At post-mortem, the cause of death is found. In addition, a 1 cm scarred area is noted in the myocardium of the lateral wall of the left ventricle.

3. How are areas of dead myocardium dealt with in the heart? What is the most common cause of myocardial scarring?

Short notes

Write short notes on the following:

1. Regeneration and repair
2. Granulation tissue formation
3. Cellular events in wound healing (skin or bone)
4. Factors affecting wound healing.

Self-assessment: answers

Multiple choice answers

1. a. **False.** Epithelioid cells and macrophage-derived giant cells are components of granulomas *not* granulation tissue. This is another common exam 'catch' question.
   b. **False.** Mast cells are involved in a variety of tissue reactions, including type 1 hypersensitivity. However, they are not essential components of granulation tissue.
   c. **True.** Granulation tissue is rich in capillaries; these channels bud off from preserved vessels adjacent to the damaged area. This process is known as neovascularisation (angiogenesis). It is probably controlled by the local production of growth factors.
   d. **True.** Fibroblasts and myofibroblasts are the other essential component of granulation tissue. These cells migrate into the damaged area and produce a variety of matrix proteins including proteoglycans, fibronectin and collagen. This process is controlled by local growth factors and cytokines. The process by which dead tissue is replaced by granulation tissue and eventually scar tissue is known as organisation.
   e. **False.** Lymphocytes are not essential to the formation of granulation tissue. However, both acute and chronic inflammatory cells can be seen in granulation tissue as it matures.

2. a. **True.** Vitamin C is required as a cofactor in collagen synthesis. A deficiency of this vitamin leads to scurvy.
   b. **False.** Lead is a heavy metal which even in small amounts is detrimental to humans.
   c. **False.** Vitamin B_{12} deficiency causes a macrocytic megaloblastic anaemia.
   d. **True.** Zinc, like vitamin C, is required for normal collagen synthesis. Zinc supplements can improve wound healing in zinc-deficient patients.
   e. **False.** It is an excess of corticosteroids (particularly corticosteroids used for the treatment of certain medical conditions) that hinders wound healing.

3. a. **False.** Labile cells are those which are capable of continuously dividing to replace themselves, e.g. bone marrow stem cells, epidermis or gastrointestinal epithelial cells. These cells are, therefore, able to regenerate when damaged. Scarring occurs after severe tissue damage (including damage to the extracellular matrix) or when permanent cells are damaged and, by definition, cannot enter the cell cycle to divide and replace themselves.

   b. **False.** Permanent cells, such as cardiac and skeletal muscle and neurones, cannot regenerate and so healing always occurs by scarring.
   c. **True.** Normal epithelial cells in culture exhibit a phenomenon known as contact inhibition. Normal cells grow in a single layer in culture and tend not to overlap or pile up on each other. If a breach is made in the layer, cell division is stimulated and the breach is healed. Cell division ceases when contact is made. This may be important in wound healing and in the uncontrolled growth of malignant cells.
   d. **True.** When damage occurs to the bowel mucosa, the cells can regenerate and heal over because they are labile. If the damage is more severe and involves the smooth muscle wall of the bowel, then healing by scarring occurs. This may narrow the lumen of the bowel and lead to a stricture and possible obstruction. Bowel cancer can also cause stricturing of the lumen.
   e. **True.** Organisation is the process whereby the body deals with inert or dead tissue. Haematoma or blood clot needs to be removed or replaced by granulation tissue before healing can take place.

Case history answers

Case history 1

1. A full thickness burn is one where the skin has been damaged right down to the subcutaneous tissue. The healing of skin wounds after burning illustrates very well how the extent of the injury to a tissue or organ influences the outcome of the repair process. In superficial burn injuries to the skin, when deeper layers of the epidermis remain intact and there is little damage to deeper adnexal structures, only a small amount of granulation tissue forms. Dead epidermis will be replaced by regeneration from adjacent viable, basal epidermal cells. A small, inconspicuous scar will eventually form. In full thickness skin burns, regeneration will be slow, granulation tissue production is extensive and often a large area of scarring will be seen.

2. Early granulation tissue (3 days to about 1 week after injury) is an oedematous mass of capillary channels and (myo)fibroblasts; acute and chronic inflammatory cells are also seen. As granulation tissue matures, the collagen content increases, reaching a maximum at about 3 to 4 weeks, and the cellular content diminishes. The capillary channels are resorbed, fibroblasts become inconspicuous and ultimately an acellular scar forms.

   The phenomenon of distorted contraction of a scar is known as cicatrisation and is particularly common in large, full thickness burns. Other complications include excessive granulation tissue production, which actually hinders wound closure (exuberant granulation) and keloid formation (abnormal amounts of scar tissue).

Case history 2

1. **Local factors**. Include here poor blood supply, difficulty in obtaining good fixation to reduce movement across the fracture site, possibly infection and foreign material in the fracture.
   Systemic factors. These are diabetes mellitus, poor cardiac function/circulation, general nutritional/health status, etc.
2. Pulmonary embolus as a result of deep vein thrombosis of the calf. Despite a variety of anticoagulation regimens in routine clinical practice to try and prevent venous thrombosis, this scenario still occurs.
3. Cardiac muscle cells are permanent cells; they are unable to divide. Dead cardiac muscle is phagocytosed by neutrophils and macrophages and granulation tissue grows in from the viable periphery. A scar eventually forms. The most common cause of myocardial infarction leading to scarring is coronary artery atheroma, with or without overlying thrombus formation.

Short notes answers

It is important to have a good understanding of these processes. It is not necessary to remember the names of all the growth factors; it is much more important to have a good grasp of the concepts of healing and repair and how the different processes are linked.

1. First define the terms 'regeneration' and 'repair' and then contrast them using examples. A simple superficial epidermal skin wound or gastrointestinal erosion will heal by regeneration because the cells are labile, whereas a deep leg ulcer or infected wound will heal by repair. Repair is the process which includes the formation of granulation tissue and then a scar.

2. Granulation tissue is a mass of new blood vessels admixed with myofibroblasts and is part of the repair process. The stages of granulation tissue formation are outlined earlier in this chapter. Use a simple diagram of wound healing to illustrate this process.

3. The cellular events in wound healing are as follows:
   a. blood clot and fibrin form a scab
   b. acute inflammatory reaction (neutrophils followed by macrophages)
   c. exudate forms, containing neutrophils, macrophages and possibly microorganisms
   d. epithelial regeneration occurs at edge of wound
   e. granulation tissue forms, i.e. new blood vessels grow in from the edges and fibroblasts and myofibroblasts migrate into the wound
   f. extracellular collagen is laid down to form scar tissue.

4. Divide the factors affecting wound healing into local (relating to the wound itself) and general (relating to the whole patient). Therefore, local factors include infection and blood supply, whereas general factors include nutritional and disease and dietary status.

Differentiation, growth disorders and neoplasia

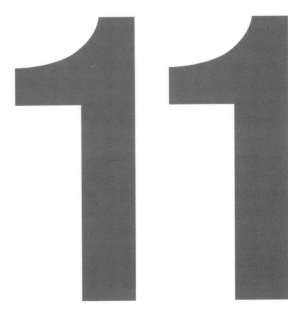

Chapter overview

Differentiation is the process by which specialised cells develop from a precursor stem cell. Hyperplasia is a physiological increase in cell number, dysplasia is a stage of disordered cell growth which may be reversible and is often thought of as pre-malignant. Neoplasia is abnormal cell growth that persists even after the inducing stimulus is removed.

11.1 Differentiation

Differentiated cells have specialised functions which are not present in the precursor stem cell. Stem cells, which have the capacity to divide continuously (labile cells) as well as produce mature cells for a given cell population, are found in most epithelial and connective tissues. Thus colonic stem cells differentiate to produce mucin-secreting cells and plasma cells produce extracellular immunoglobulin, which is not seen in lymphoid stem cells. Maintenance of the differentiated state is controlled by the genetic programming of the cell and the local environment in which it grows (systemic hormones, local growth factors and matrix proteins). Although each somatic cell contains the whole potential human genome, groups of genes can be switched on or off. If this control system goes wrong, differentiation and functional specialisation may not occur. This loss of differentiation is seen in the early stages of cancer formation.

Hyperplasia

Hyperplasia is enlargement of a tissue or organ by multiplication of cell number (see chapter 3). This is normally physiological and reversible. For example, the proliferative endometrium of the uterus in the first half of the menstrual cycle is stimulated by oestrogen. If the endometrium is stimulated by large amounts of inappropriate oestrogen produced by an ovarian cancer, the resulting hyperplasia may persist and become pathological; ultimately neoplasia (cancer) may occur.

Dysplasia (disordered growth)

Dysplasia is a condition of disordered cell growth and proliferation which may arise de novo or from tissues already showing pathological hyperplasia (atypical hyperplasia), metaplasia, or chronic inflammation/irritation. Early stage dysplasia may be reversible if the stimulus is removed but may also progress to become neoplasia (cancer).

Clinical pathology of dysplasia and neoplasia

In many clinical situations, we recognise that there is a spectrum of change from hyperplasia to dysplasia and finally to neoplasia. In practice it is very difficult to identify absolute cut off points between these growth disorders. Identification of epithelial dysplasia clinically is usually regarded as a pre-malignant change and treated accordingly.

Neoplasia

What is cancer and how does it develop? Neoplasia literally means 'new growth'. A variety of terms are used to describe the phenomenon of neoplasia: neoplasm, tumour (which actually means a swelling) and cancer/carcinoma are often used synonymously. This may cause confusion. A neoplasm is an abnormal tissue mass which grows in an uncoordinated way and persists after the inducing stimulus (if known) has been removed. This autonomous growth is usually detrimental to the host. Malignant neoplasms may spread to sites distant from the original area of growth (metastasis/secondary deposits). Neoplastic cells usually resemble their normal counterparts but may lose all their differentiating features so that the tissue of origin cannot be identified (anaplasia). The microscopic features of neoplastic cells may be identical to those listed below for dysplasia.

It is possible to grow neoplastic cells in culture in the laboratory. As a result of such work, several important differences in the growth behaviour of neoplastic cells compared with normal cells have been identified.

Neoplastic cells show:

- **transformed phenotype** (Fig. 26), which means that they may:
  — not require extrinsic growth factors
  — proliferate to form colonies (clones)
  — show reduced cell cohesiveness
  — show altered surface antigens
  — grow to higher cell densities in a haphazard way
  — not show normal cell orientation
- **tumorigenicity**, which means that they will grow into tumours when injected into immunosuppressed animals
- **immortality**, which means that they can undergo indefinite replication and can be grown as cell lines.

Mechanisms of invasion and metastasis

Many cancer cells produce enzymes such as collagenases, which are proteases that digest various forms of collagen. This and other matrix-degrading enzymes help tumour cells to invade adjacent tissues. Normal tissue produces protease inhibitors, which may be neutralised by tumour cells. These properties are seen in tumours which behave aggressively.

The ability of a neoplasm to metastasise is what distinguishes a benign tumour from a malignant tumour. Metastasis is the seeding of tumour cells to sites distant and detached from the original one. Cells can spread to distant sites via the bloodstream or lymphatics, or across body cavities. The exact mechanism whereby

A Normal

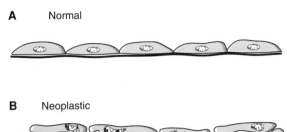

B Neoplastic

Fig. 26
Growth of normal versus neoplastic cells.

tumour cells will start to grow in a distant site is not known. Survival and growth of metastases depend on the local environment and seem to be helped by the presence of platelets and production of platelet-derived growth factor (PDGF). Tumour cells may have cell adhesion molecules or binding sites which enable them to 'home' in on the endothelia of particular tissues.

Dysplasia/neoplasia

The position of dysplasia as a potential transition stage in the development of true neoplasia is supported by a number of clinical situations where the sequence appears defined. Dysplasia and neoplasia have some common features and show a progression from normal cell character to the neoplastic state.

Microscopic features of dysplasia/neoplasia

These are:

- loss of normal maturation pattern (polarity)
- increased mitotic figures (some may be atypical)
- variation in cell shape and size (pleomorphism)
- large nuclei in relation to cytoplasm
- dark staining nuclei (hyperchromatism as a result of increased DNA content)
- cells may look more 'primitive' (altered differentiation).

When there is complete loss of polarity of an epithelium which is composed entirely of dysplastic cells, the term 'carcinoma in situ' (CIS) is used. Penetration by dysplastic cells through the basement membrane of the epithelium is not seen — the abnormal cells are confined to the epithelium. Increasingly severe dysplasia with CIS formation can often be seen close to a cancer which is obviously invading local tissues. This is circumstantial evidence that cancers may evolve from dysplastic lesions.

Recognition that dysplasia is a pre-malignant condition forms the basis of screening for some types of cancer. An important example of this is the **cervical smear test**, designed to identify clusters of cells with nuclear and cytoplasmic changes which correlate with changes in the intact epithelium known as CIN (cervical intra-epithelial neoplasia). Appropriate treatment can then be given to prevent the development of invasive cervical cancer, e.g. laser or cryotherapy to the abnormal area.

Clinical examples of the dysplasia to neoplasia sequence

1. **Benign colorectal polyps** (adenomas) are actually composed of dysplastic epithelial glands. If left in situ, without treatment, the majority of these will turn into malignant neoplasms over the course of several years (Fig. 27). Familial adenomatous polyposis (FAP) is an inherited (autosomal dominant) disease in which hundreds and

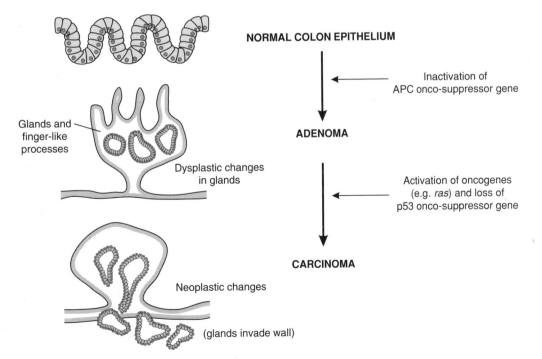

Glands and finger-like processes

Dysplastic changes in glands

Neoplastic changes

(glands invade wall)

NORMAL COLON EPITHELIUM

Inactivation of APC onco-suppressor gene

ADENOMA

Activation of oncogenes (e.g. *ras*) and loss of p53 onco-suppressor gene

CARCINOMA

Fig. 27
The adenoma–carcinoma sequence.

thousands of adenomas develop in the colon. These all have malignant potential and the colon must be removed prophylactically, i.e. to prevent colon cancer occurring.

2. Identification of dysplasia in the uterine cervical epithelium is the beginning of a spectrum of changes known as cervical intraepithelial neoplasia (CIN), which if untreated will develop into malignant neoplasia.

3. Atypical hyperplasia, dysplasia and carcinoma in situ in female breast epithelium are not usually detected clinically but may be diagnosed using mammography, which forms part of the breast-screening programme. Such lesions are considered to be pre-malignant and may warrant treatment to prevent the onset of breast cancer.

11.2 Carcinogenesis

Carcinogenesis is the process which results in the development of a malignant neoplasm (cancer) (Fig. 28). Cells may undergo neoplastic transformation as a result of a series of discrete genetic changes, or mutations. The risk of a mutation increases with the number of mitotic divisions experienced by a cell, so that labile tissues tend to be more prone to neoplastic change than stable or permanent ones.

A carcinogen is a substance which can cause neoplasia by its action on nuclear DNA (Table 14). Many carcinogens require cofactors which are not themselves capable of producing neoplastic change but which have a cumulative or synergistic effect with the carcinogen. There may be a long latent interval between exposure to the carcinogen and development of cancer. Carcinogenesis is a multistep process which requires the action of an initiating agent followed by promoting factors acting on the cells.

Oncogenes

Molecular biology techniques have revolutionised our understanding of the role of genes in cancer development. The critical mutations which are caused by carcinogens are now known to occur within a set of well defined cancer-related genes (oncogenes). Some of these human DNA sequences (proto-oncogenes) bear striking similarities to known cancer-causing genes in certain viruses (viral oncogenes) and many normally control cell proliferation.

Cellular oncogenes are sequences of DNA in the human genome which when extracted and injected into a cultured cell can cause neoplastic transformation.

Dysplasia

Neoplasia

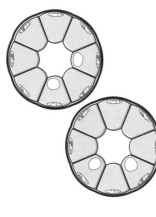

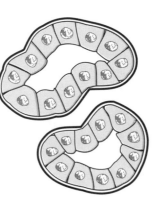

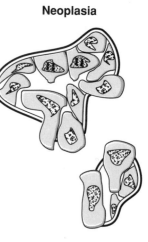

Normal colonic gland	Dysplastic colonic gland (adenomatous)	Neoplastic colonic glands (adenocarcinoma)
Basal nuclei	Larger non basal nuclei	Irregular shapes and sizes
Regular shape and size	Irregular size	Large nuclei
Goblet cell differentiation	Loss of polarity	Mitotic figures
	Confined to gland basal membrane	Cells invade outside basal membrane
	Loss of goblet cell differentiation	

Fig. 28
Carcinogenesis.

Table 14 Examples of known carcinogens

Carcinogen group	Examples	Cancer
Chemicals	Polycyclic hydrocarbons Azo dyes	Lung cancer (smoking) Bladder cancer
Viruses	Hepatitis B virus Human papilloma virus	Liver cancer Cervical cancer
Ionising radiation	X-rays Uranium/radon Radioactive iodine	Skin cancer Lung cancer Thyroid cancer
Non-ionising radiation	UV light	Malignant melanoma (skin cancer)
Hormones	Anabolic steroids	Liver cancer
Toxins	Aflatoxins	Liver cancer
Parasites	Liver fluke	Bile duct cancer
Industrial dust	Asbestos	Malignant pleural tumour (mesothelioma)

Proto-oncogenes do not normally cause transformation but when **activated** by changes in adjacent genes or in themselves may lead to mutation. This means that the proto-oncogene may be **amplified**, with multiple copies causing excessive production of gene product (i.e. growth factors). Alternatively, chromosomal translocation may place the proto-oncogene next to a normally distant DNA sequence which then causes activation. Integration of tumorigenic viruses into human DNA may cause activation of proto-oncogenes in a similar way.

Onco-suppressor genes

These are genes which appear normally to prevent neoplasia. Therefore, if these genes are inactivated, then the individual is predisposed to cancer. In human cancer families where there is a familial tendency to develop cancer, the genetic abnormalities seem to involve inactivation of the normal suppressor gene.

Examples of onco-suppressor genes

The best described are the *RB-1* gene for familial retinoblastoma and the *APC* gene in familial adenomatous polyposis (FAP). Another anti-oncogene codes for a protein called p53, which has roles in regulating cell proliferation and triggering apoptosis and is increasingly being recognised as an important factor in many neoplastic growths by stopping mutated, potentially cancerous, cells from entering the cell cycle and dividing (see Fig. 27 and Fig. 28).

Epidemiological factors

There are many well recognised epidemiological factors which are associated with the development of cancer:

- genetic and cultural factors: stomach cancer is very common in Japan, much less so in the UK

- diet: smoked and preserved foods are linked to gastric cancer
- gender: male more than female in many cases which affect both sexes (e.g. rectal cancer)
- family history: breast and colon cancer in first-degree relatives
- pre-malignant conditions: ulcerative colitis, undescended testis
- fetal exposure: maternal stilboestrol treatment leading to vaginal cancer in female offspring.

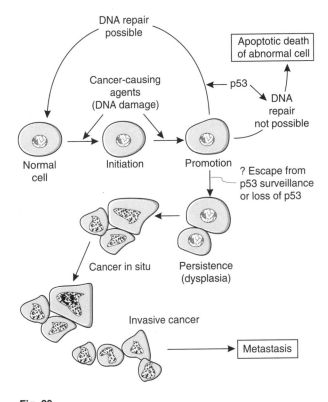

Fig. 29
Control of DNA damage.

Self-assessment: questions

Multiple choice questions

1. Dysplastic epithelium:
   a. Inevitably becomes neoplastic
   b. Characteristically shows lack of polarity
   c. May show nuclear pleomorphism
   d. May occur in metaplastic epithelium
   e. In the cervix may be detected by a smear

2. Oncogenes:
   a. May be present in normal cells
   b. Are produced by activation of proto-oncogenes
   c. Cannot be detected in histological preparations
   d. Produce mutant oncoproteins
   e. Resemble RNA retrovirus particles

3. The following are correctly paired:
   a. Dysplasia — irreversible
   b. Hepatitis B virus — liver cancer
   c. X-rays — cell cytoplasm damage
   d. Asbestos bodies — mesothelioma
   e. UV light — skin cancer

Case history

A 74-year-old man is admitted to hospital with a cough which is sometimes bloodstained, breathlessness and weight loss. A chest X-ray shows a shadow in the upper part of the left lung. Sputum is sent to the pathology laboratory for examination of any cells coughed up. The pathologist's report says 'numerous severely atypical (dysplastic) squamous cells seen'.

1. What is meant by dysplasia? What microscopic features of the cells would lead the pathologist to this diagnosis?

A piece of tissue (biopsy) is taken from the area of lung shadowing and this shows a malignant neoplasm (carcinoma). The lung is removed surgically. When samples are taken from the bronchial epithelium adjacent to the cancer, squamous metaplasia is seen.

2. Define metaplasia. Give three examples.
3. How might the normal–tissue-metaplastic tissue–neoplastic tissue sequence occur?

Short notes

1. Compare and contrast the cellular features of dysplasia and neoplasia.
2. Discuss occupational cancers.

Self-assessment: answers

Multiple choice answers

1. a. **False.** The progression of dysplasia to neoplasia is controversial. It is probable that mild forms of dysplasia are completely reversible.
   b. **True.** In dysplasia, even mild forms, loss of epithelial organisation and stratification occur.
   c. **True.** Nuclear pleomorphism — varying shapes and sizes of nuclei — is typical of dysplasia. This phenomenon often becomes more pronounced the more severe the dysplasia becomes.
   d. **True.** Metaplasia and dysplasia often occur together, e.g. Barrett's metaplasia of the oesophagus is a condition in which the squamous lining of the oesophagus is replaced by intestinalised, glandular epithelium probably as a result of chronic inflammation. Patients with this condition are at risk of developing dysplastic and then neoplastic changes if not treated.
   e. **True.** Detection of epithelial dysplasia by cervical smears is the basis of the screening programme for cervical cancer.

2. a. **True.** Oncogenes are pieces of DNA which are present in all cells and normally are responsible for the regulation of cell growth. Their transcription is tightly controlled. In neoplastic growth, the normal oncogene control mechanisms become deranged.
   b. **True.** The proto-oncogene or normal cellular oncogene may be uncovered, activated or amplified, leading to uncontrolled growth of the cell. The *myc* and *ras* oncogenes are good examples of oncogenes which have well-characterised effects in the early stages of tumorigenesis.
   c. **False.** Using molecular biology techniques, it is possible to apply DNA probes for various oncogenes to tissue sections of normal and neoplastic tissues. This enables the pathologist to visualise the distribution of the expression of oncogenes.
   d. **True.** When an oncogene is 'switched on' this may result in the production of an abnormal gene product or, alternatively, increased amounts of a normal protein product. Oncoproteins are involved in the regulation of cell proliferation, growth factors, growth factor receptors and intracellular signalling mechanisms.
   e. **True.** Oncogenic RNA viruses are retroviruses that produce reverse transcriptase and have been known to be capable of producing tumours experimentally for many years. It was then realised that normal DNA contains sequences which are identical to some of these RNA viruses.

3. a. **False.** Dysplasia is essentially a reversible (adaptive) process particularly in its mild forms. However, it is difficult to know exactly when it changes to the irreversible process of neoplasia. Many dysplastic lesions will progress to cancer if left untreated.
   b. **True.** Hepatitis B virus is strongly associated with the development of liver cancer. The virus inserts its DNA into the hepatocyte DNA. In the Far East, HBV infection is endemic and liver cancer is very common.
   c. **False.** X rays are known to be important initiators of many types of cancer. The cell damage is directed at the nucleus and causes genetic mutations in the cells.
   d. **True.** Asbestos fibres are inhaled and can produce lung fibrosis (asbestosis). They can also lead to the development of malignant mesothelioma (a pleural cancer). Most asbestos exposure is occupational and people who have worked in docks, lagging ships' boilers, are at high risk of mesothelioma. There is often a long lag period between the time of exposure and onset of tumour. This may be as long as 20–25 years.
   e. **True.** UV light is associated with the development of malignant melanoma and squamous cell carcinoma, as well as with many kinds of benign proliferative skin lesions. UV light causes damage to cellular DNA, leading to mutations.

Case history answer

1. A succinct definition of dysplasia is difficult. Literally, it means perverted growth! Atypical hyperplasia is also a term used, which can be confusing. Dysplasia encompasses a constellation of histological and cytological features, including loss of polarity and tissue organisation as well as cytological signs of abnormal growth and maturation (nuclear pleomorphism and increased numbers of mitoses).
2. Metaplasia is easier to define. The 'reversible, adaptive change from one adult cell type to another adult cell type in a tissue' is adequate. Remember that although metaplasia most often occurs in epithelial systems, connective tissues can also undergo metaplasia (e.g. osseous metaplasia). When you are asked for examples of metaplasia think of hollow viscera that may become inflamed or obstructed. The chronically inflamed, transitional epithelium of the urinary bladder (which may also contain stones) will often show areas of squamous metaplasia. In most examples of epithelial metaplasias, specialised cells such as the pseudo-stratified, ciliated columnar respiratory epithelium

of the bronchus undergo metaplasia to a less specialised, basic cell type (squamous cells). This is almost certainly because, in the face of a continuing, adverse environment caused by inhaled cigarette smoke, squamous cells are more resilient and do not have to maintain specialised functions. When the noxious stimulus is removed (patient gives up smoking!), the epithelium can revert to its more sensitive, specialised form.

3. There is much research into this area of cell biology. It is likely that in most cases metaplasia is gene mediated. Therefore, certain novel genes are switched on in the labile stem cells replenishing an epithelium exposed to an adverse environment. The new cells will have a different complement of intracellular and surface proteins. If the noxious stimulus continues or increases, the new cell type may also be affected and the genome begins to acquire mutations; ultimately a neoplastic clone may grow out of the epithelium.

Short notes answers

1. There are some similarities and some differences between dysplasia and neoplasia. Define both the terms at first, stressing the irreversible nature of neoplasia and the reversible nature of (at least mild forms of) dysplasia. Use a clinical example such as CIN and cervical carcinoma.

2. Give one or two examples of occupational cancer (mesothelioma in dock workers, skin cancer in early radiologists) and then indicate what the carcinogen is thought to be and how it fits into the multistep theory of carcinogenesis. Distinguish between initiators and promoters.

Classification
of neoplasms

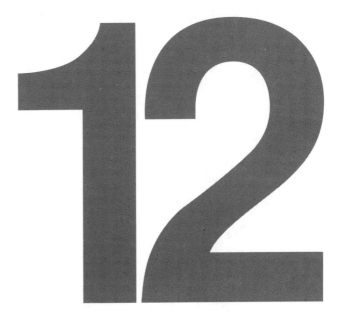

Chapter overview

In the USA and UK the highest death rates are from cancer arising from the lung in men, the breast in women and the colon/rectum in both men and women. Skin cancers of all kinds are increasing in incidence in the Western world. The death rates from cancer do not necessarily reflect their incidence, i.e. skin cancer is common but easily treated at an early stage, so that the mortality is low. Breast cancer is also common but has a high death rate.

12.1 Growth of neoplasms

Wherever a tumour develops, it needs a blood supply and supporting matrix. All neoplasms develop their own fibrovascular stroma which sustains the nutrition and growth of abnormal cells. Tumours commonly undergo necrosis when their rate of growth exceeds the capacity of the stroma to provide sustenance.

Neoplasms show a variety of growth patterns, depending on their site of origin, speed of growth and cellular characteristics (Fig. 30):

- ulcerating
- polypoid
- exophytic.

Behaviour of tumours

Neoplasms can behave in a benign or malignant way. The main distinction between a benign and a malignant tumour is that benign tumours do not metastasise (i.e. spread by the bloodstream or lymphatics to other parts of the body). That does not mean to say that a benign tumour cannot grow aggressively or, by virtue of its position and local effects, kill the patient (e.g. a benign tumour in a vital area of the brain can be inoperable and ultimately lethal).

Benign neoplasms tend to show the following features:

- localised growth which is confined to the tissue of origin
- well circumscribed or encapsulated
- slow growing (low mitotic rate)
- well differentiated, i.e. resemble the tissue of origin
- no distant spread (metastasis)
- cause symptoms by local effects, e.g. pain/pressure/obstruction/hormone production.

Malignant neoplasms tend to show the following features:

- invade the tissue of origin
- can metastasise
- metastases cause cachexia (generalised body wasting) and anaemia
- may arise de novo or from a pre-existing benign neoplasm
- tend to be poorly circumscribed (often do not have a capsule)
- fast growing and aggressive
- show poor differentiation (may not resemble tissue of origin)
- cause local symptoms such as pain
- cause symptoms according to their site, e.g. coughing blood with lung cancer.

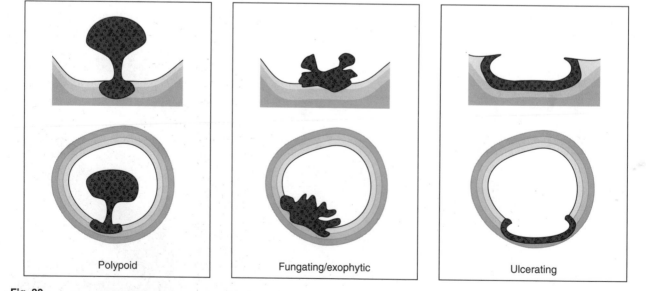

Fig. 30
Patterns of neoplastic growth.

Polypoid | Fungating/exophytic | Ulcerating

12.2 Spread of neoplasms

Benign tumours do not spread beyond their site of origin. They may grow to be extremely large and may distort or disrupt local tissues, but they never spread to distant sites. Malignant neoplasms, however, show several different modes of spread. This starts locally. Most carcinomas spread initially via the lymphatics and metastasise to the local draining lymph nodes (lymphatic spread). In advanced carcinomas and most sarcomas, distant spread occurs via the bloodstream (haematogenous spread).

Local invasion. Cervical cancer will eventually invade the urinary bladder and ureters. Gastric cancer may invade through to the pancreas.

Metastasis:

- direct seeding, e.g. transcoelomic (across the peritoneal cavity) spread of colorectal cancer in the abdomen
- lymphatic spread, e.g. axillary lymph node involvement in breast cancer; inguinal lymph node involvement in a malignant melanoma of the skin of the leg
- haematogenous spread, e.g. liver involvement via portal venous system in gastric cancer; bone metastases from breast cancer.

The most common sites for blood-borne metastases are bone, lung, brain and liver.

12.3 Nomenclature of neoplasms

Neoplasms are named according to their tissue of origin and nearly all have the suffix '-oma' (Table 15). Malignant neoplasms arising from epithelial tissues are called carcinomas and those arising from mesenchymal tissue are called sarcomas (Fig. 31).

A hamartoma is a non-neoplastic lesion which is composed of a mixture of tissues normally found at the site and grows slowly with the host. For example, hamartomatous polyps of the bowel consist of smooth muscle, glandular elements and blood vessels. Bronchial hamartomas contain cartilage, smooth mus-

Table 15. Examples of the nomenclature of neoplasms

Tissue of origin	Benign	Malignant
Squamous epithelium	Papilloma	Squamous carcinoma
Glandular epithelium	Adenoma	Adenocarcinoma
Smooth muscle	Leiomyoma	Leiomyosarcoma
Fat	Lipoma	Liposarcoma
Bone	Osteoma	Osteosarcoma
Skeletal muscle	Rhabdomyoma	Rhabdomyosarcoma

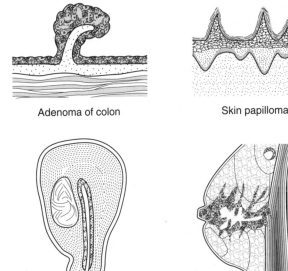

Adenoma of colon

Skin papilloma

Uterine fibroid (leiomyoma)

Carcinoma of breast

Fig. 31
Examples of benign and malignant tumours.

cle and bronchial epithelium. Whether these are true tumours or malformations is hotly debated.

A teratoma is a neoplasm which is derived from tissues of more than one germ cell layer (and usually all three layers — endoderm, mesoderm and ectoderm).

Staging and grading of neoplasms

It is important to be able to predict the clinical outcome of a neoplasm. The grade of a neoplasm is related to a combination of histological factors, including cellular differentiation, mitotic and apoptotic rate and the amount of necrosis present. The stage of a neoplasm is determined by how far it has spread at the time of diagnosis. Good examples of prognostic staging are the Dukes' staging system for colorectal cancer (Fig. 32) and the use of Breslow's thickness (the depth of invasion) in malignant melanoma (see the box on the next page). In general, the better differentiated the neoplasm and the earlier it is detected and treated, the better the outlook for the patient.

There are a number of factors that determine prognosis in addition to tumour grade and stage:

- site (suitability for surgery, etc.)
- patient's age (and general health)
- responsiveness to treatment particularly important in lymphomas and leukaemias (tumours of the lymphoid and blood cell systems).

Screening

Because most invasive malignant neoplasms arise as a result of a sequence of cellular events which cause normal cells to transform into neoplastic ones, there is often a stage at which they are clinically pre-malignant, i.e. non-invasive. In practice, this means that the tissues show fea-

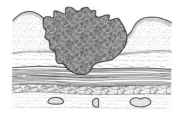

Dukes A

Tumour confined to bowel wall

Good prognosis

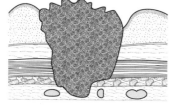

Dukes B

Tumour invades through the bowel wall

Intermediate prognosis

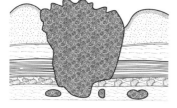

Dukes C

Lymph node metastasis

Poor prognosis

Fig. 32
Dukes' staging of colorectal cancer.

tures of dysplasia or carcinoma in situ, a term which describes carcinoma confined to an epithelial surface with no evidence of local or other spread. Many epithelial neoplasms can be detected early in their development. It is important to detect cancers early, because with appropriate treatment, the neoplasm can be removed before it metastasises and kills the patient. This principle forms the basis of cancer screening programmes.

Screening procedures currently available are:

- cervical smear—uterine cervical cancer
- mammography—breast cancer (see the box on page 109)
- endoscopic removal of adenomas colorectal cancer
- skin surveillance for pigmented tumours malignant melanoma.

Malignant melanoma

- Increasing in incidence in the Western world
- Affects young and middle-aged adults
- Risk factors:
  — fair skin
  — existing atypical moles (dysplastic naevi)
  — exposure to sunlight (short sharp bursts)
- Signs: pigmented skin lesions which increase in size, itch, bleed, are ulcerated, or are irregularly pigmented
- Diagnosis: clinical suspicion and biopsy
- Origin: melanocytes in the basal layer of the epidermis become neoplastic and proliferate upwards and outwards (radial growth) or downwards into the dermis (vertical growth)
- Prognosis: as long as the melanoma is confined within the epidermis and is in a radial growth phase, there is a good prognosis. Once the neoplasm has spread into the dermis, it has metastatic potential and, therefore, a worse prognosis.

  Pathologists always measure the maximum depth of invasion of a melanoma (Breslow's thickness), which correlates well with survival. Thus the 5-year survival of patients with tumours less than 0.76 mm thick is 98% whereas with tumours more than 1.5 mm thick it decreases to 50%
- Staging:
  I   localised skin tumour only
  II regional lymph node metastases, i.e. groin nodes for leg lesions, cervical lymph nodes for head and neck lesions
  III distant metastases via the bloodstream occur in the liver, brain and lungs and sometimes unusual sites such as bowel and heart.

Tumour markers

Some tumours produce substances which can be detected in the blood or urine (or tissue itself by immuno-histochemistry) and can be used in the diagnosis or monitoring of the neoplasm. The substances may be normal products produced in excessive amounts or abnormal substances usually only seen in primitive or fetal tissues (Table 16).

Table 16 Tumour markers

Marker	Tumour
Carcinoembryonic antigen (CEA)	Colorectal disease, benign and malignant
Human chorionic gonadotrophin (HCG)	Malignant teratoma
Alpha-fetoprotein (AFP)	Malignant teratoma, hepatoblastoma
Prostatic acid phosphatase	Prostate cancer
Vanillyl mandelic acid (VMA)	Neuroblastoma
5-Hydroxy indole acetic acid (5HIAA)	Carcinoid tumour

Breast cancer

- Most common malignancy in women in the Western world
- 50% overall mortality rate
- Risk factors:
  — increasing age
  — strong family history (genetic factors)
  — increased oestrogen exposure
  — early menarche
  — late menopause
- Protective factors:
  — early first pregnancy
  — oophorectomy under 35 years of age
- Screening:
  — self-examination
  — mammography
- Diagnosis:
  — mammography
  — fine needle aspiration cytology
  — biopsy
- Prognosis:
  — size of tumour: early detection of small tumours with treatment gives a better prognosis
  — lymphatic invasion: breast carcinoma like most epithelial tumours metastasises via the lymphatics to local lymph nodes, in this case the axillary nodes. The more nodes involved and the higher up the axilla (i.e. further away from the primary tumour) they are, the worse the prognosis
  — tumour differentiation: poorly differentiated tumours which barely resemble the tissue origin (i.e. the breast duct or lobule) have a worse prognosis.

Self-assessment: questions

Multiple choice questions

1. The following are correctly paired:
   a. Carcinoma of breast — malignant proliferation of breast stroma
   b. Osteosarcoma — malignant proliferation of bone marrow cells
   c. Familial Retinoblastoma — tumour of the eye in elderly people
   d. Large bowel obstruction — colonic carcinoma
   e. Meningioma — tumour of cerebral cortex

2. The following statements are true:
   a. Of people with Dukes' stage A carcinoma of the rectum, 90% will survive for 5 years
   b. Lipomas are common benign tumours of fat
   c. Poorly differentiated carcinomas usually have a poor prognosis
   d. Most carcinomas initially metastasise via the regional lymph nodes
   e. Leukaemia is a malignant neoplasm arising from the peripheral white blood cells

Case history

A 53-year-old woman presented to her doctor with a lump in her breast. On examination, the lump was in the upper outer quadrant of the right breast and was fixed to the skin which was puckered over the surface. The nipple was slightly inverted. The lump felt hard and craggy to palpation and was approximately 4 cm in diameter. The GP felt several enlarged lymph nodes in the axilla on the same side. The patient admitted that the lump had been present for at least a year, but she had been too scared to see her doctor before.

The GP referred her urgently to a breast surgeon. Fine needle aspiration with examination of the cells removed showed that the tumour was malignant and surgery was performed (lumpectomy with axillary node clearance). The pathologist reported that the tumour was a malignant carcinoma of ductal origin which had been completely excised. The lymph nodes contained metastatic tumour.

Several months later the patient presented with pain in the femur and a pathological fracture.

1. Why was the lump fixed to the skin?
2. How does breast cancer spread?
3. What might have been the outcome if the patient had been to her doctor when she first noticed the lump?
4. What is the significance of the bone pain and fracture?
5. Name some of the known risk factors for breast cancer.

Short notes

Write short notes on the following:

1. Principles of screening for cancer
2. Dukes', staging of colorectal cancer.

Essay question

1. What are the important macroscopic and microscopic features of neoplasms which determine the outcome for the patient?

Self-assessment: answers

Multiple choice answers

1. a. **False.** Carcinoma of the breast is the most common tumour in women of the Western world and arises from a malignant proliferation of the epithelium of the ducts and/or lobules. Malignant proliferations of breast stroma are extremely rare and are called breast sarcomas.

   b. **False.** Osteosarcoma is a malignant neoplasm of the bone-producing cells (osteoblasts). Bone marrow cells are part of the lymphoreticular and haematopoietic system and give rise to lymphoma and leukaemia.

   c. **False.** Familial Retinoblastoma is a rare malignant tumour of the retina which is inherited as an autosomal recessive condition. Both copies of part of chromosome 13 are deleted. Therefore, the tumour develops shortly after birth and is only seen in infants and babies. In general, most cancers are commoner in the elderly than in the very young.

   d. **True.** Colorectal adenocarcinoma commonly grows into the lumen of the bowel in an exophytic fashion. As the tumour becomes more advanced, it invades locally through the bowel wall and can form a circumferential constriction which leads to obstruction. The constriction may be visualised through the endoscope or on barium radiograph where a characteristic 'apple core' feature is seen.

   e. **False.** Meningioma is a benign neoplasm of the meninges, usually the dura mater. The lesion is usually well differentiated, well circumscribed and can be successfully removed surgically. However, the site of the lesion is crucial because as it enlarges it may press on vital structures and cause severe disability or even death.

2. a. **True.** Dukes' stage A carcinoma is confined to the bowel wall and hence its capacity for metastasis is limited. Patients with this early stage of cancer, therefore, have a good prognosis, provided the tumour is completely eradicated.

   b. **True.** Benign fatty tumours are very common. Malignant fatty tumours are very rare and are called liposarcomas.

   c. **True.** In general, the less well differentiated a tumour is, the worse its prognosis. There are, however, other important factors which determine prognosis and which may override the grade of tumour. These are stage, size, site, patient's age and responsiveness to treatment.

   d. **True.** Lymph node spread forms the basis of most staging systems. The following are common:

- carcinoma of bronchus—hilar lymph nodes
- breast carcinoma—axillary lymph nodes
- carcinoma of the perineum—inguinal lymph nodes
- testicular cancer—para aortic lymph nodes.

   e. **False.** Leukaemia is a malignant proliferation of bone marrow stem cells, which are the precursors of mature leucocytes. The type of leukaemia depends on the clone of stem cells which are affected. Therefore, there are leukaemias of lymphocytes, granulocytes, monocytes.

Case history answer

1. Tumour fixation indicates that the tumour was invading local structures of the breast, which include not just the adjacent breast tissue but the overlying skin. This gives it a puckered appearance. Sometimes tumour cells obstruct the lymphatics of the overlying skin, resulting in oedema and pitting of the surface rather like the skin of an orange. This clinical sign is called 'peau d'orange' and is a bad prognostic sign.

2. Breast cancer follows the general rules of spread of all cancers. Firstly, local structures such as the skin and nipple may be involved. As the tumour develops, it spreads via the lymphatics to draining lymph nodes, in this case to axillary lymph nodes on the same side. Eventually, haematogenous spread may occur with seeding of tumour to the bones, lung, brain or liver.

3. If the patient had presented earlier, there would have been a chance that the tumour had not already spread either so extensively locally or to the lymph nodes. The earlier tumours are detected, usually, the better the prognosis. Breast screening programmes should reduce the death rate from breast cancer.

4. The bone pain is caused by metastatic breast carcinoma (haematogenous spread) which has invaded the femur and caused it to become weak and fracture spontaneously (pathological fracture).

5. There is no single risk factor for breast cancer but it is more common in women who have had an early menarche or had their first child late (see the box on breast cancer, p. 109). The converse seems to be true, i.e. women who have their first child at a younger age have a reduced risk. Breast feeding may be protective and there is no evidence that the contraceptive pill increases the risk. Smoking and some dietary factors may increase the risk and genetic factors are important in some cases, where the disease may run in families. Some women who have a strong family history of breast cancer appear to have inherited a mutant gene or genes (e.g. BRCA 1 and 2). These genes give an increased susceptibility to developing breast cancer.

Short notes answers

1. The principles of cancer screening depend on pathological and epidemiological information. Therefore, a knowledge of the biological behaviour of the disease is essential. This includes growth rate, mode of spread and risk factors to identify appropriate target groups for screening. Any screening test must be:

   - reliable and sensitive, i.e. always pick up positive cases and not lead to false negatives
   - specific, i.e. only diagnose the disease for which it is intended
   - acceptable to the public, i.e. relatively non-invasive (see Ch. 1).

2. The best way to answer this question would be to outline the survival rates for each given stage and use a diagram to illustrate the invasion of the tumour and how it spreads.

Essay answer

1. This question is all about the staging and grading of malignant tumours. It is important to show an understanding of the way in which tumours behave and grow at the tissue and cellular levels.

   At the cellular level the important points are: (i) neoplastic cells have certain biological characteristics which differentiate them from normal cells, i.e. uncontrolled growth; (ii) histological features such as differentiation (how much the tumour cells resemble their tissue of origin), mitotic activity and apoptosis/necrosis (an indication of cell turnover and how fast the tumour is growing in relation to its stroma and blood supply) all give some indication as to the grade of tumour. It is a general principle that tumours which are at the better end of this spectrum may behave in a less aggressive fashion.

   Macroscopically, the growth of tumours and how they spread is important for identifying the stage of tumour, i.e. has it just invaded locally or have tumour cells seeded into the lymphatic or blood systems. The Dukes' staging system is a good model for the staging of most neoplasms and could be used as an example in this essay.

   Another aspect which you could bring in to the discussion is that of the early detection of cancer and the principles upon which this is based.

Cell and tissue degeneration and accumulation

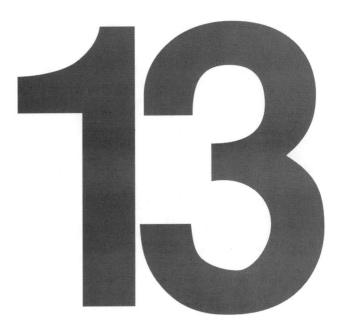

Chapter overview

There are several important pathological entities or processes that do not fit neatly into the classical categories of disease. Amyloid is a good example of this and is a favourite examination topic, especially in MCQs and vivas. In clinical practice (particularly renal medicine) amyloid is more common than might be expected. It is, therefore, important to have a working knowledge of this interesting entity. Degeneration and calcification are probably less important from an exam point of view; they are, however, referred to in textbooks and so are dealt with briefly in this chapter.

13.1 Degeneration

The term 'degeneration' was used to describe a variety of pathological processes. Formerly, the term was widely used in relation to cell injury. Thus, 'feathery' and 'fatty' degeneration were used to describe the appearance of reversibly injured cells. The term 'feathery' is now little used and fatty degeneration is more appropriately called fatty change.

Nowadays, degeneration is used to describe pathological processes which result in deterioration (often with destruction) of tissues and organs. Therefore, osteoarthritis is an example of degenerative joint disease in which gradual destruction and deterioration of the bones and joints occurs. Alzheimer's disease is an example of a degenerative neurological disease where there is a progressive deterioration in brain function. Other pathological terms in skin and renal pathology imply degeneration of tissues. An example would be UV-induced degeneration of the connective tissue in skin: solar elastosis.

13.2 Accumulation

Cells may accumulate pigments or other substances as a result of a variety of different pathological or physiological processes. The accumulations can be classified as endogenous or exogenous.

Fatty change

Fatty change represents accumulation of triglyceride in cells and is usually an early indicator of cell stress and reversible injury. The most common cells in which fatty change is seen are in the liver, which has a central role in fat metabolism. Excessive alcohol consumption is a common cause of this, but there are other causes. In the liver, fatty accumulation occurs when cell damage compromises the ability of the hepatocyte to bind fat to protein and transport it through the cell. Fatty change is

also seen in cardiac muscle cells as a result of severe anaemia or starvation (anorexia nervosa).

Haemosiderin

Haemosiderin is a golden yellow to brown pigment found in lysosomes within the cell cytoplasm. It is composed of aggregates of partially degraded ferritin, which is protein-covered ferric oxide and phosphate. When there is an excess of iron, e.g. when there is a breakdown of red blood cells or haemorrhage, haemosiderin accumulates in cells. It can be visualised using the Prussian blue reaction, when haemosiderin appears dark blue.

Primary haemochromatosis is an inherited disease in which there is excessive accumulation of iron and widespread deposition of haemosiderin in the tissues, especially the liver, pancreas and skin. The iron is toxic to the tissues and leads to fibrosis of the liver (cirrhosis) and pancreas (leading to diabetes mellitus).

Melanin

Melanin is the brown/black pigment which is normally present in the cytoplasm of cells in the basal layer of the epidermis, called melanocytes. Melanin is derived from tyrosine, stored in melanosomes and distributed to the other epidermal cells. The function of melanin is to block harmful UV rays from the epidermal nuclei. Melanin may accumulate in excessive quantities in benign or malignant melanocytic neoplasms and its presence is a useful diagnostic feature melanocytic lesions. In inflammatory skin lesions, where the epidermis is damaged, melanin may be released from injured basal cells and taken up by dermal macrophages. This gives rise to post-inflammatory pigmentation of the skin. Melanin can be identified in tissue sections by the use of the Masson–Fontana stain.

Lipofuscin

This is the yellow/brown wear-and-tear pigment seen in atrophic tissues, particularly in heart muscle (see Atrophy, Ch. 3).

Other pigments and dyes

Pigments and insoluble substances may enter the body from a variety of sources. They may be toxic and produce inflammatory tissue reactions or they may be relatively inert. Indian ink pigments produce effective tattoos because they are engulfed by dermal macrophages which become immobilised and permanently deposited. Inhaled substances such as coal dust and silica are engulfed by pulmonary macrophages. Although pure carbon is inert, silica and coal dust are toxic and ultimately cause serious lung fibrosis (pneumoconiosis).

Calcification

There are two main types of calcification:

- dystrophic
- metastatic.

Dystrophic calcification

This type of calcification occurs within diseased tissues. The plasma calcium and phosphate levels are normal. The exact mechanism by which dystrophic calcification occurs is not known. The best examples include calcification within foci of old tuberculosis and in atheromatous plaques. In both these cases, the calcification can often be seen, incidentally, on radiographs.

Metastatic calcification

Metastatic calcification often occurs in normal tissues as a consequence of raised plasma calcium concentrations (hypercalcaemia). Common causes of hypercalcaemia include widespread metastatic cancer in the bones (bony metastases), hyperparathyroidism and multiple myeloma.

Amyloidosis

The term 'amyloid' means 'starch-like' and as such is misleading because amyloid is not a carbohydrate. Amyloid is a descriptive term used for a group of proteinaceous substances that may deposit in tissues and organs to give characteristic naked eye, microscopic and ultrastructural appearances.

What is amyloid?

The type of protein found in the amyloid deposits depends on the underlying disease. For example, in patients with multiple myeloma (a neoplastic proliferation of antibody-producing plasma cells), the amyloid is composed of antibody fragments. Whatever the main constituent protein, the amyloid deposit also contains a second substance, a glycoprotein known as the P component (or P protein). The main protein is always deposited as long, non-branching fibrils (these can be seen under the electron microscope and have a diameter of about 8 nm). The P component is a doughnut-shaped pentamer. It is the fibrillar protein and the P component that account for some of the interesting properties of amyloid:

- when deposited in tissues in large amounts the tissue becomes pale, smooth and waxy in texture
- histologically, amyloid stains pink with congo red dye; the pink colour turns apple green under polarised light, a property unique to amyloid

- by X-ray crystallography, amyloid has a beta-pleated sheet conformation
- the body's intra- and extracellular proteolytic enzyme systems find amyloid almost impossible to 'digest'; therefore, there is an inexorable accumulation of amyloid, which may compromise the function of the organ involved.

Where does amyloid accumulate?

Amyloid can accumulate within any tissue or organ. The disease may affect just one tissue/organ — localised amyloidosis — or several — systemic amyloidosis. It always accumulates outside cells and has a predilection for basement membranes and interstitial connective tissues. Where there is abundant amyloid deposition, cells become 'strangled' and organ failure occurs.

When does amyloid accumulation occur?

There are two important clinical situations in which amyloid deposition occurs and the form of amyloid differs in the two.

AL amyloid. Patients with multiple myeloma (a neoplasm of plasma cells) have excessive amounts of circulating intact and fragmented immunoglobulin. Complete or fragmented light chains can produce amyloid light chain (AL amyloid).

AA amyloid. The second type of amyloid complicates long-term inflammatory conditions. These can be pus-forming processes, such as bronchiectasis where pus accumulates in dilated airways in the lung, or autoimmune diseases, such as rheumatoid disease (see Ch. 8). In these conditions, the liver produces a number of so-called 'acute phase proteins'. Amongst these is serum amyloid A protein (SAA) which produces amyloid A (AA amyloid).

Other amyloids. There are numerous other proteins which can produce amyloid, such as pre-albumin (transthyretin), calcitonin and β_2-microglobulin, but these are rare.

What are the effects of amyloid on tissues/organs?

This will depend on the organs involved. A localised deposit of amyloid may cause no problems and only be discovered incidentally, e.g. localised amyloid of the bladder during the course of X-ray examination of the urinary tract. Renal involvement can lead to the loss of large amounts of protein in the urine and even renal failure. Myocardial amyloid may stop the heart contracting properly or, if deposited in the conducting system, cause a lethal arrhythmia.

Self-assessment: questions

Multiple choice questions

1. The following are correctly paired:
   a. Lipofuscin pigment — tattoos
   b. Haemosiderin pigment — skin bruising
   c. Congo red stain — amyloid
   d. AL amyloid protein — bronchiectasis
   e. Parathyroid adenoma — hypercalcaemia

2. The following statements are true:
   a. Fatty change caused by alcoholic liver damage is reversible
   b. Lipofuscin accumulation is associated with ageing
   c. Calcification of atherosclerotic plaques is rare
   d. Anthracosis is caused by silica
   e. Epidermal cells take up pigments in a tattoo

Case histories

Case history 1

A 56-year-old woman presented with generalised symptoms of feeling unwell. She had noticed swelling of her ankles and face and was breathless. On examination, she was noticed to have signs of heart failure and oedema. Her urine, collected over 24 hours, contained 11 g of protein (normal is less than 150 mg) and her serum albumin level was 20 g/l (normal is about 40 g/l).

A kidney biopsy was performed and showed amyloid deposition. Further examination of the urine and serum proteins showed increased amounts of lambda light chain proteins. Bone marrow biopsy showed an increased number and proportion of plasma cells which were all producing the same type of immunoglobulin molecule (monoclonal proliferation).

1. What is multiple myeloma and how does it produce amyloidosis?
2. How does amyloidosis affect the kidney?
3. How can amyloid be diagnosed in tissues?
4. Why might the loss of large amounts of protein in the urine lead to ankle swelling?

Case history 2

A 58-year-old accountant was noticed by his family and firm to have become unreliable, mentally slow, confused and have a poor memory. Over the next few years, he became progressively unable to walk and lead an independent existence. He died at the age of 67. Clinically, a diagnosis of Alzheimer's disease was made during his illness.

1. What is Alzheimer's disease?
2. Why does the study of Down's syndrome sufferers help us in the understanding of Alzheimer's disease?

Short notes

Write short notes on the following:

1. Fatty change
2. Haemosiderin
3. Melanin
4. Amyloid.

Viva questions

1. What are the causes of hypercalcaemia?
2. What is the difference between dystrophic and metastatic calcification?
3. What types of amyloid do you know of?

Self-assessment: answers

Multiple choice answers

1. a. **False.** Lipofuscin is the brown intracellular pigment which is found in cellular atrophy. It is present in autophagic vacuoles within cells and is often known as wear-and-tear pigment. Organs which are very atrophic may actually look brown to the naked eye from excessive amounts of this pigment. Tattoos gain their colour and permanence from the intradermal injection of inks and dyes, often based on carbon or mercury pigments. These are ingested by local macrophages which cannot digest them and become immobilised at the site of the tattoo, the colour remaining visible through the skin.
   b. **True.** Haemosiderin is the iron-based pigment resulting from the breakdown of haemoglobin. When haemorrhage occurs into tissues, red cell haemoglobin is degraded and ingested by macrophages. Haemosiderin is a brownish yellow pigment which gives the bruise its characteristic colour.
   c. **True.** Congo red stain is a useful diagnostic test for the presence of any type of amyloid within the tissues. Amyloid stains salmon pink with congo red and shows apple green birefringence under polarised light.
   d. **False.** AL amyloid is composed of kappa or lambda immunoglobulin light chains and is found in amyloid derived from immunoglobulin, most commonly in multiple myeloma. Multiple myeloma is a neoplastic monoclonal proliferation of plasma cells which produces abnormal amounts of a single immunoglobulin. Bronchiectasis leads to chronic infection of the lungs which can lead to AA protein amyloid formation.
   e. **True.** Parathyroid adenoma is a benign tumour of the parathyroid glands which can produce abnormal amounts of parathyroid hormone. This leads to increased levels of calcium in the bloodstream (hypercalcaemia), which causes fits, vomiting and excessive urine production (polyuria), and sometimes metastatic calcification.

2. a. **True.** Fatty change is a reversible degenerative process. It is most commonly seen in the liver and the heart. Fatty change occurs as a result of sublethal injury. In the liver, intracellular triglycerides must be complexed with protein in order to transport them through the cell. Alcohol interferes with this metabolic process and hence causes fatty change.
   b. **True.** Lipofuscin is associated with ageing and can be seen accumulating in many major organs

in elderly people. Lipofuscin itself is not injurious to cells.
   c. **False.** Calcification of atherosclerotic plaques is a very common condition. It is caused by dystrophic calcification.
   d. **False.** Anthracosis is caused by the accumulation of carbon pigment in lung macrophages. It is seen in coal miners and city dwellers.
   e. **False.** The tattoo pigments are taken up by dermal macrophages which stay in place for ever.

Case history answers

Case history 1

1. Multiple myeloma is an uncontrolled proliferation of plasma cells. It is characterised by excessive production of immunoglobulin, usually IgG or IgA or light chains. The onset of the disease may be very gradual and the patient may not experience symptoms until it has caused complications such as kidney disease or hypercalcaemia as a result of bone destruction. The light chains deposit in the kidney or form amyloid protein (AL amyloid), which deposits in many organs, especially the kidneys, heart and gut.
2. Amyloid deposits mainly in the walls of blood vessels, basement membranes and intercellular areas. Therefore, in the kidney, amyloid will affect blood vessel walls, which may lead to ischaemia of the kidney. Deposits in the tubular basement membrane lead to failure of resorption of water and electrolytes, and deposition in the glomerular basement membrane leads to protein loss in the urine.
3. Tissues which contain abundant amyloid will stain dark blue-black when iodine is poured on them and sulphuric acid added. Under the microscope, amyloid is best visualised using the congo red stain and looking for the characteristic pink staining and green birefringence under polarised light. Electron microscopy will reveal the characteristic tangle of non-branching amyloid fibrils.
4. Protein loss in the urine leads to a reduced intravascular colloid osmotic pressure and hence hydrostatic pressure forces fluid out of the blood vessels into the interstitium. This is clinically seen as tissue oedema.

Case history 2

1. Alzheimer's disease is the most common primary dementia. It is more common in women than men. At autopsy, the brain is atrophic and often weighs less than 1000 g whereas a normal adult brain would weigh 1200–1400 g. Microscopically, there is

an overall loss of neurones. Those that remain show bundles of abnormal filaments in their cytoplasm (neurofibrillary tangles). The characteristic neuritic plaques which are present are composed of masses of filaments surrounding an amyloid core. Amyloid may also be present in the walls of cerebral blood vessels. The cause of Alzheimer's disease is not known. It has been likened to 'accelerated ageing'.

2. Patients with Down's syndrome (trisomy 21) who survive to middle age show similar neuritic plaques and neurofibrillary tangles in their cerebral cortex. Therefore, it has been postulated that genes on chromosome 21 may play an important role in the development of these degenerative changes in Alzheimer's disease.

Short notes answers

1. Fatty change results from many kinds of sublethal cell injury and leads to the accumulation of fat droplets in the cell cytoplasm. Organs affected by fatty change appear enlarged, pale and have a greasy consistency. Fatty change commonly occurs in the liver, where it is a feature of liver cell damage caused by drugs or alcohol. Fat accumulation also occurs in starvation where protein deficiency results in a reduced capacity for the protein binding and transport of triglyceride out of cells.

2. This iron-rich protein is seen in histological sections as a golden brown pigment. Haemosiderin is seen in tissue when there is a breakdown of haemoglobin either following trauma or as a result of iron overload from blood transfusion or injected iron treatment. Haemosiderin may accumulate in tissues such as the liver where it is ingested by liver macrophages (Kupffer cells) or in the bone marrow or spleen macrophages.

3. Melanin is a sulphur-containing iron-free pigment. It is dark brown in colour and is formed in melanosomes, mainly in skin melanocytes. Extracellular melanin is taken up by macrophages.

Melanin pigment may be altered in a variety of conditions:

- UV light stimulates melanin (suntanning)
- vitiligo is a condition where there is patchy loss of melanin
- pigmented tumours may be benign (pigmented naevi) or malignant (malignant melanoma).

4. Amyloid is a proteinaceous deposit in tissues and organs that has a characteristic appearance although the type of protein depends on the underlying disease. Because amyloid is hard to break down it continues to accumulate and may compromise function. Discuss the structure and components of amyloid, the clinical situations in which it occurs and its effects on the functions of tissues and organs.

Viva answers

1. The causes of hypercalcaemia are numerous. In order to approach this question sensibly and give the most important causes, think about the mechanisms which might bring this about. For example:

- high calcium intake: dietary
- increased resorption of calcium from bones: bony metastases, renal disease
- increased production of parathyroid hormone: parathyroid adenoma, some types of lung cancers
- abnormal vitamin D, calcium and phosphate: renal disease
- artefactual; excess venous stasis at venesection.

2. Define the terms 'dystrophic' and 'metastatic' and give examples of both. Be prepared to go on to talk about mechanisms of hypercalcaemia.

3. Define the term 'amyloid'. Name the two important forms of amyloid, AA and AL, and describe how they are formed and how they differ. Again, give clinical examples.

Glossary

ADCC (antibody-dependent cell-mediated cytotoxicity)
A cytotoxic reaction where Fc receptor-bearing killer cells recognise target cells via specific antibodies.

Adenocarcinoma
A carcinoma derived from glandular epithelium, e.g. adenocarcinoma of colon.

Adenoma
A benign tumour of glandular epithelium.

Allergen
An agent that causes IgE-mediated hypersensitivity reactions, e.g. pollen, house dust mite.

Allergy
Common term for a type 1 hypersensitivity reaction.

Alternative pathway
The complement cascade, which is triggered by a variety of factors such as tissue damage and starts with C3.

Anaemia
A reduction in the oxygen-carrying capacity of the blood, almost always the result of abnormalities of red cells, e.g. iron deficiency, premature destruction (haemolysis) and abnormal haemoglobins.

Anaphylaxis
The antigen-specific immune reaction mediated by IgE which results in systemic vasodilatation and constriction of smooth muscle (including those of the bronchus), leading to shock and sometimes death.

Anoxia
Complete loss of oxygen supply, often the result of obstruction of blood supply.

Antibody
A molecule produced by B cells (plasma cells) in response to antigen with which it can specifically bind.

Antigen
A molecule which reacts with preformed antibody on B cells and T cell receptors.

Antigen-presenting cells (APCs)
These can process and present antigen to lymphocytes. Examples are the dendritic cells of the lymph nodes, and the Langerhan's cells of the skin.

Apoptosis
A form of programmed individual cell death which occurs normally during embryological development. It also occurs in pathological processes such as atrophy and neoplasms. It is an energy-dependent process which is not associated with an inflammatory reaction.

Atrophy
The gradual loss of an organ or tissue because of either natural ageing (e.g. gonads) or a pathological process (such as ischaemia).

Atypia
Changes in the histological appearance of cells, usually suggesting neoplastic transformation. Very similar meaning to dysplasia.

Autolysis
The changes that occur in an organ or tissue after removal from the body, and in the whole body after death. No vital (inflammatory) reaction seen.

Basophil
Basophilic polymorphonuclear leucocytes. A white blood cell with a multi-lobated nucleus and coarse cytoplasmic granules. Comprises 1% of the total white cell count in peripheral blood.

Biopsy
A procedure which removes a sample of cells or tissues for histological examination by a pathologist. Usually performed during life.

Blood group, blood group antigen
The result of the expression of an antigen at the red cell membrane. There are many different 'groups' but the most important in clinical practice are the ABO and the rhesus systems.

BCG (Bacille–Calmette–Guérin)
An attenuated strain of *Mycobacterium tuberculosis* used as a vaccine.

Cachexia
The term used to describe the clinical appearance of a patient with advanced cancer. There is often marked weight loss and the patient is 'emaciated' and wasted. Probably cytokine-induced.

Cancer
A lay term used to describe any form of malignant tumour.

Carcinogenesis
The process/processes by which neoplasms develop. Often qualified by the causative agents, e.g. viral carcinogenesis, chemical carcinogenesis.

Carcinoma
A malignant tumour derived from epithelial tissue.

Carcinoma in situ
An epithelial neoplasm with all the histological and biological characteristics of malignancy but which has not (yet) invaded through the basement membrane. Best known example is cervical intraepithelial neoplasia (CIN).

Carcinomatosis
Carcinoma in many different organs following extensive metastases from a primary tumour.

CD markers
Cluster differentiation markers are molecules on leucocytes, platelets and other cells that can be recognised with monoclonal antibodies and may be used to differentiate different cell populations.

Cell cycle
The process of cell division which comprises four phases: G_1, S, G_2, and M. DNA replicates in the S phase and the cell divides in the M (mitotic) phase. A further phase, G_0, contains cells that are no longer dividing.

Cell death
'The point of no return'. The transition between non-lethal and lethal cell injury.

Cell injury
The consequence of a wide variety of different insults, e.g. bacteria, viruses or physical agents. Can be lethal (causing cell death) or non-lethal (producing degenerative changes).

Cell-mediated immunity
Immune reactions which are mediated by cells (lymphocytes) rather than antibody.

Chemotaxis
The purposeful movement of cells (neutrophils, macrophages) in response to a chemical stimulus.

Classical pathway
The pathway by which antigen–antibody complexes can activate the complement system, involving complement proteins C1, C2 and C4.

Clone
A family of cells which is genetically identical.

Clot
An ill-defined term. In *lay usage* a thrombus, but *strictly* the appearance of blood in the body after death (post-mortem clot). Blood tends to sediment in vessels after death forming a plasma-rich 'jelly' (chicken fat clot) and dark masses of red cells.

Complement
C1–C9 are the serum protein components of the complement cascade which are responsible for mediating inflammatory reactions, opsonisation of particles and cell lysis. The cascade can be activated by the immune system (classical pathway) or by tissue damage (alternative pathway).

Cyclosporin A
A T cell-suppressive drug which is useful in the suppression of graft rejection.

Cytokines
A family of messenger proteins which stimulates the maturation or activation of a variety of cells including lymphocytes and macrophages. These were originally known as lymphokines, when it was thought they were only secreted by lymphocytes. They have wide variety of different physiological and pathological effects, including the maturation of haemopoietic stem cells.

Degeneration
The changes which follow non-lethal cell injury.

Dysplasia
Changes in the histological appearance of cells which indicate that they have become, or may become, neoplastic. Best described in the squamous epithelium of the skin, cervix and bronchus.

EBV (Epstein–Barr virus)
Causal agent of Burkitt's lymphoma (a malignant proliferation of immortalised B cells) and infectious mononucleosis (glandular fever).

Embolus
Material which circulates in the blood and lodges in a blood vessel and occludes it. Examples of emboli are air, thrombus, fat and amniotic fluid.

Emigration
The process by which inflammatory cells leave blood vessels and enter the tissue.

Endocytosis
The physiological mechanism by which fluid is taken in small discrete amounts into the cell cytoplasm from the interstitial tissues.

Eosinophil
Eosinophilic polymorphonuclear leucocyte. A white blood cell, often with a bilobed nucleus and eosinophilic (intensely pink) cytoplasmic granules. They have many functions, including breakdown of histamine and killing of parasites. Comprise 2–3% of total white cell count in peripheral blood.

Epithelioid cell
A macrophage commonly found in tuberculous lesions. In histological preparation, these cells have eosinophilic cytoplasm and superficially resemble epithelial cells — hence their name.

Exudate
An abnormal collection of fluid within tissues, or in a body cavity. The protein concentration of an exudate is usually high and there is almost always associated inflammation.

Fatty change (fatty degeneration)
A potentially reversible form of cell injury, most often seen in the liver. The result of impaired cytoplasmic metabolism of fat.

Gangrene
A characteristic 'blackening' of necrotic tissue. Produced by infection with anaerobic bacteria and tends to occur in tissues which have a resident bacterial flora, e.g. skin and large bowel.

Giant cell
A large cell with many nuclei. In chronic inflammation, giant cells are formed by the fusion of macrophages. These must be distinguished from tumour giant cells — cancerous cells with a bizarre histological appearance.

Granulation tissue
The richly vascular tissue containing inflammatory cells and myofibroblasts which is laid down in the first stages of repair.

Granuloma
A localised aggregate of macrophages and other inflammatory cells. There are many examples of 'granulomatous diseases' including tuberculosis, leprosy, schistosomiasis and Crohn's disease.

Growth factors
Polypeptides which stimulate protein synthesis within individual cells. Attach to specific receptors on the cell surface. Are involved in cell proliferation. Good examples include PDGF (platelet-derived growth factor) and epidermal growth factor.

Healing by primary intention
The normal process by which surgical wounds heal. The close apposition of the edges of the wound is essential and only small amounts of granulation tissue are laid down.

Healing by secondary intention
The process by which large wounds whose edges cannot be apposed heal. There is abundant granulation tissue formation and a large amount of scarring.

Hyperplasia
The increase in the size of an organ or tissue as a result of an increase in the number of constituent cells. Can only occur in labile or stable tissues, i.e. tissues which can undergo mitotic division.

Hypertrophy
The enlargement of a tissue or organ resulting from an increase in the size of the constituent cells, *not* an increase in number. Examples include cardiac hyper-trophy in hypertension and skeletal muscle in athletes.

Hypoxia
A shortage of oxygen, but not an absolute lack (anoxia).

Infarct
An area of necrosis produced by an obstruction of the circulation.

Inflammation
A mechanism by which the living body reacts to many different forms of injury. Acute inflammation has both vascular and cellular components and usually lasts for days or a few weeks. In chronic inflammation, there is mixed cellular response, including macrophages and cells derived from macrophages, and the process can last for months or years.

Initiator
The first step in the two-step theory of carcinogenesis. This postulates that an initial change, probably some form of genetic alteration (mutation), is followed by a second step, promotion. This theory is supported by several well-described experimental models of chemical carcinogenesis but is probably oversimplistic, even for those human tumours produced by environmental agents.

Ischaemia
Shortage of blood flow, often a result of an obstruction to the circulation.

Immune complex
The product of an antibody–antigen reaction, which may also contain components of complement.

Interferons/interleukins
A group of molecules involved in signalling between cells of the immune system, also known as cytokines or lymphokines.

Küpffer cells
Phagocytic macrophages which line the liver sinusoids.

Lymphoma
Malignant tumour of lymphoid tissue or macrophages. Chiefly involves lymph nodes, spleen and bone marrow but can affect many other organs.

Lysosomes
Cytoplasmic organelles completely enclosed by membranes and containing a wide variety of enzymes. The release of these enzymes after cell death in living tissue produces some of the changes of necrosis.

Macrophage
A mononuclear cell derived from blood monocytes with phagocytic properties. Prominent in the chronic inflammatory response.

Margination
The process by which inflammatory cells come to lie at the margins of blood vessels, just before emigrating to the adjacent tissue. A characteristic feature of acute inflammation. Mediated by adhesion molecules.

Mediator
A chemical substance which instigates, or controls, a physiological or pathological response — the best known mediators are those which modulate the inflammatory reaction (e.g. histamine).

Metastasis
Transfer of tumour from one site (the primary) to another (the secondary), usually via the blood or lymphatic systems. Defines a malignant tumour.

Monocyte
A mononuclear white blood cell, derived from precursors in the marrow. After migration into the tissues they are known as macrophages or histiocytes.

Myofibroblast
A specialised cell characteristically seen in granulation tissue. The cytoplasm of these cells contains contractile filaments and they are largely responsible for closing up the gap between the edges of wounds.

MHC (major histocompatibility complex)
A genetic region primarily responsible for the rapid rejection of grafts between individuals. In the human the MHC is also known as the HLA.

Necrosis
The changes which occur in organs or tissues after cell death in a living body. Often taken to include cell death.

Neoplasm
A 'new growth' of tissue. In common usage a tumour, either benign or malignant.

Neutrophils
Neutrophil polymorphonuclear leucocytes. The commonest form of white cell in the blood (about 50–60% of the total) actively phagocytic, important in the acute inflammatory response.

Oedema
The accumulation of abnormal amounts of fluid in tissue. Occurs when the normal balance between the hydrostatic pressure of the circulation and the osmotic force of the plasma proteins is upset.

Oncogene, proto-oncogene, viral oncogene
An oncogene is a gene which codes for a protein that contributes to the tumorous characteristic ('phenotype') of a neoplastic cell. They are related to, and probably derived from, proto-oncogenes, which have important roles in normal cellular physiology, especially in the control of 'cell growth'. Viral oncogenes are fragments of genetic material carried by viruses into normal cells, which then influence the expression of the tumorous phenotype. In both humans and animals, proto-oncogenes are given short code names: *ras*, *myc*, *erbB*, *sis*, *abl*.

Oncoproteins
The proteins encoded by 'oncogenes'. The functions of a few of these are now partially understood. Some can mimic the action of growth factors.

Opsonisation
A process whereby phagocytosis is helped by the coating of antigen with antibody and/or complement (C3b).

Pathogen
An organism which causes disease.

Phagocytosis
The process by which material is ingested by specialised inflammatory cells (polymorphs, macrophages, giant cells and eosinophils).

Phagosome
The 'bag' of inverted cell membrane enclosing the phagocytosed material or particle.

Promoter
The second stage in the two-step theory of carcinogenesis (initiator — promoter). Could involve a wide range of different agents, e.g. hormones, nutritional state, ageing, immunological status.

Putrefaction
The process of decomposition of animal or vegetable matter by living organisms (usually bacteria or insects). Often has an associated foul odour.

Pyknosis
The dark condensed appearance of the nucleus of a dead cell undergoing necrosis. May eventually fragment (karryorhexis) or wither away (karryolysis).

Regeneration
The proliferation of a labile or stable tissue (e.g. bone marrow stem cells, kidney or liver cells) in an attempt to restore that tissue to normality. In clinical practice, most injuries are followed by both regeneration and repair.

Repair
The process by which a tissue defect is replaced with scar tissue. In most areas of the body this is fibrous tissue, although in the brain glial tissue (gliosis) is laid down.

Sarcoma

A malignant tumour derived from mesenchymal tissue (e.g. fibrous tissue: fibrosarcoma; bone: osteosarcoma; adipose tissue: liposarcoma).

Scar

A dense mass of fibrous tissue (collagen) laid down to repair a defect when regeneration is not possible.

Stem cell

A primitive haemopoietic cell capable of maturation into a variety of different mature forms. The most primitive is the pluripotent stem cell, which first matures into lymphoid or myeloid stem cells.

Teratoma

Tumour with elements derived from all three germ layers — often arises in ovary (usually benign) or testis (usually malignant).

Thrombus, thrombosis

An aggregate of platelets and fibrin with enmeshed leucocytes. Only forms in living vessels with flowing blood. Sometimes has a banded light and dark appearance (lines of Zahn). They may fragment and embolise (thrombo-embolism).

Translocation

The transfer of a gene from its normal position to one on another chromosome. Occurs regularly in some tumours (e.g. chronic myeloid leukaemia and Burkitt's lymphoma), involving sites of chromosomes occupied by proto-oncogenes. The rearrangement of these segments is, therefore, a key step in the development of the tumorous characteristics.

Transudate

An accumulation of fluid with a low protein content in the tissues or the body cavity. In contrast to an exudate, there is usually no associated inflammation — the fluid usually accumulates because of circulatory factors.

Tuberculosis

A chronic inflammatory disorder produced by infection with mycobacteria. The classical disease involves the lungs and can spread to many other organs. Result of infection with *Mycobacterium tuberculosis*.

Ulcer, ulceration

A localised area of loss of the epithelium and underlying tissues (cf. erosion — only the epithelium is lost). Many different causes including inflammation (inflammatory ulcer) and tumour (neoplastic or malignant ulcer).

Index

Note: Question and Answer Sections are indicated in the form 14Q/16A

A

Abscess, 84Q/85A
Acquired diseases, 5, 6Q/9A
ADCC, 64, 119
Adenocarcinoma, 119
Adenoma, 119
Adenoma-carcinoma sequence, 99-100
Adhesion molecules, 80, 81
Aetiology, 4-5, 6Q/9A
Agammaglobulinaemia, Bruton's, 73
AIDS, 73-74, 75Q/77A
Allergen, 119
Allergy, 119
Alternative pathway, complement system, 40, 41, 119
Alzheimer's disease, 116Q/117-118A
Amyloid, 115, 116Q/118A
Amyloidosis, 115, 116Q/117A
Anaemia, 119
Anaphylatoxins, 41
Anaphylaxis, 43, 70, 119
Anaplasia, 98
Aneurysm, 49
Ankylosing spondylitis, 64
Anoxia, 119
Antibody, 58, 59, 64, 65Q/66A, 119
    classes and functions, 60
    diversity, 59, 65Q/68A
    structure, 59-60
    see also Antigen-antibody complexes
Antibody-dependent cell-mediated cytotoxicity (ADCC), 64, 119
Antibody response, 61-62, 65Q/67A
Antigen, 58-59, 119
Antigen-antibody (immune) complexes, 40, 41, 61, 71, 75Q/76A
Antigen-presenting cells (APC), 61, 62, 65Q/66A:67A, 119
Antigenic determinants, 58-59
Antigens, 61, 63-64
Apoptosis, 31-32, 34Q/35A, 119
Appendicitis, 84Q/85A-86A
Arthus reaction, 71
Asthma, 70, 75Q/76A:77A
Atherosclerosis, 48-49, 52Q/53A:54A
    complications, 48-49
    pathogenesis, 48
    risk factors, 48, 52Q/54A:55A
Atrophy, 21-22, 24Q/25A:26A, 119
Atypia, 119
Autoantibodies, 72
Autoimmune disease, 59, 72, 75Q/77A
Autolysis, 31, 34Q/35A:36A, 119
Autopsy, 12, 16Q/18A

B

B cells, 58, 59-60, 61, 62, 64, 65Q/66A:67A
Basophils, 80, 119
BCG, 119
Biliary cirrhosis, 72
Biopsy, 12, 119
Blood clotting, 40, 41-42, 44Q/45-46A, 49-50, 52Q/54-55A
Blood group/blood group antigen, 119
Blood transfusion, incompatible, 70
Bone fracture healing, 91, 93Q/95A
Bone marrow, 58
Bradykinin, 40
Breast cancer, 109, 110Q/111A
    screening, 100
Bruton's agammaglobulinaemia, 73

Burn healing, 90-91, 92, 93Q/94-95A

C

Cachexia, 119
Calcification, 115, 116Q/118A
    atherosclerotic plaque, 49
Cancer, 119
    apoptosis and, 31-32
    cells, 98-99
    metastasis, 98-99, 107, 110Q/111A
    nomenclature, 107-108, 110Q/111A
    occupational, 102Q/104A
    prognosis, 108, 110Q/111A:112A
    screening, 99, 100, 108, 110Q/112A
    spread, 107
    staging and grading, 107-108
    tumour growth, 106
Carcinogenesis, 5, 100-101, 119
Carcinogens, 100, 101
Carcinoma, 107, 119
Carcinoma in situ (CIS), 99, 119
Carcinomatosis, 120
Cardiac muscle cells, 24Q/25A
Cascade systems, 40
CD markers, 61, 62, 65Q/66A:67A, 120
Cell adhesion molecules (CAM), 80-81
Cell-mediated immunity, 61-63, 65Q/67A, 120
Cells
    accumulation, 114-115
    adaptation, 20, 21-23
    cycle, 20-21, 24Q/25A:26A:27A, 120
    death, 31-33, 34Q/35-37A, 120
    degeneration, 5, 114
    immune system, 56
    inflammation, 5, 80-81, 84Q/86A
    injury, 30-31, 34Q/35A:36A, 120
    labile, 20, 24Q/27A, 98
    neoplastic, 98
    normal growth, 20-21, 24Q/26A
    permanent, 20, 24Q/27A
    regeneration, 20, 24Q/27A, 90, 93Q/95A
    repair, 20, 24Q/27A, 90, 93Q/95A
    stable, 20, 24Q/27A
Cervical intraepithelial neoplasia (CIN), 99, 100
Cervical smear test, 99
Chemotaxis, 80, 84Q/85A:86A, 120
Cholesterol and atherosclerosis, 48, 52Q/53A
Classical pathway, complement system, 40, 41, 120
Classification, 5
Clone, 120
Clostridia spp., 32
Clot, 120
Cluster differentiation molecules, 61, 62, 65Q/66A:67-68A, 120
Coagulation, 40, 41-42, 44Q/45-46A, 49-50, 52Q/54-55A
    disseminated intravascular, 42, 44Q/45A
Coagulopathy, consumption, 42
Collagen
    blood clotting, 41, 44Q/45A
    chronic inflammation, 82
    healing, 20, 90, 91
Colon, adenoma-carcinoma sequence, 99-100
Colony-stimulating factors, 63
Colorectal cancer, Dukes' staging system, 108, 110Q/111A:112A
Complement system, 40-41, 44Q/45A, 64, 120

Congenital diseases, 5, 6Q/8A
Cyclins, 21
Cyclosporin A, 120
Cystic fibrosis, 6Q/8A
Cytokeratin, 14, 16Q/17A
Cytokines, 61, 63, 64, 65Q/67A, 82, 120
Cytology, 12

D

Degeneration, 5, 114, 120
Diabetes mellitus, type I, 72
Diagnosis, 12, 16Q/17A
    differential, 12
    role of pathologist, 12-15
Diapedesis, 81, 84Q/85A
DiGeorge's syndrome, 73
Disease
    aetiology, 4-5, 6Q/9A
    classification, 5
    definition, 4
    epidemiology, 4
    health, illness and, 4-5, 6Q/7A
    idiopathic, 5
    pathogenesis, 5, 6Q/9A
Disseminated intravascular coagulation (DIC), 42, 44Q/45A
DNA-RNA-protein pathway, 14, 15
Dot blot analysis, 14
Dyes, accumulation in tissue, 114-115
Dysplasia, 98, 102Q/103A:104A, 120
    neoplasia and, 99-100

E

Electron microscopy, 12, 16Q/18A
Embolism, 50, 51, 52Q/53A:54A
Embolus, 120
Emigration of cells, 81, 120
Endocytosis, 120
Endonuclease, 31
Endoplasmic reticulum, hypertrophy, 22
Endothelium, role in clotting, 40, 41
Endotoxin, 40, 41
Eosinophils, 80, 120
Epidemiology, 4
Epithelioid cells, 63, 83, 120
Epstein-Barr virus (EBV), 120
Examinations, 1-2
Exudate, 81, 84Q/85A, 120

F

Factor VIII, 44Q/45A
Factor XII (Hageman factor), 40, 42, 44Q/45A
Familial adenomatous polyposis (FAP), 99-100, 101
Fat necrosis, 32
Fatty change, 114, 116Q/118A, 120-121
Fibrin, 40, 41-42, 44Q/45A, 81, 84Q/85A, 90
Fibrinogen, 41-42, 44Q/45A
Fibrinolysis, 40, 42, 50
Fibroblasts, 90, 91
Fish oils, 48
Free radicals, 30, 34Q/35A:37A
Frozen sections, 12, 16Q/17A

G

Gangrene, 32-33, 34Q/35A:36A, 52Q/54A, 121
Gas gangrene, 32
Gastrointestinal tract, healing, 91
Gene probes, 14
Genetic diseases, 5, 6Q/7A
Giant cells, 83, 84Q/85A:86A, 121

Granulation tissue, 82, 90, 91, 93Q/94A:95A, 121
Granulomas, 63, 83, 121
Graves' disease, 72
Growth factors, 21, 24Q/25A, 48, 121

H
Haematoxylin and eosin (H&E) stain, 12
Haemochromatosis, primary, 114
Haemolytic disease of newborn, 71, 75Q/77A
Haemophilia, 44Q/45A
Haemosiderin, 114, 116Q/118A
Haemostasis, 40, 41-42, 44Q/45-46A
Hageman factor (Factor XII), 40, 42, 44Q/45A
Hamartoma, 107
Hay fever, 70
Healing, 90-91, 93Q/95A
  bone fractures, 91, 93Q/95A
  by first (primary) intention, 90, 93Q/95A, 121
  by secondary intention, 90-91, 121
  factors affecting, 90, 93Q/94A:95A
  gastrointestinal tract, 91
Hepatocytes, 20, 22, 24Q/25A
Histamine, 70, 80, 82, 84Q/85A
Histology, 12
HIV infection, 73-74
HLA system, 63-64
Hybridisation, in situ, 14, 16Q/17A
Hypercalcaemia, 115, 116Q/118A
Hyperplasia, 21, 22, 24Q/25A:26A, 98, 121
Hypersensitivity, 70-72
Hypersensitivity reactions, 75Q/76A:77A, 80
Hypertrophy, 22, 24Q/25A:26A, 121
Hypoxia, 30, 121

I
Idiopathic disease, 5
Illness, definition, 4
Immune complex diseases, 71, 75Q/76A
Immune complexes, 40, 41, 61, 71, 75Q/76A, 121
Immunity/immune response, 5, 58-64
  adaptive, 58-59, 65Q/68A
  cellular, 61-63, 65Q/67A
  humoral, 59-61, 65Q/67A
  innate, 58, 65Q/68A
  natural defences, 58-59
  overview, 64
  properties of immune response, 58-59
Immunodeficiency, 73-74
Immunoglobulin(s), 14, 59, 60, 65Q/66A:67A
Immunohistochemistry, diagnostic, 13-14
Immunoperoxidase technique, 13, 14, 16Q/17A
Incidence of disease, 4, 6Q/8A:9A
Infarct/infarction, 34Q/37A, 51, 52Q/53-54A, 121
Inflammation, 5, 121
  acute, 81-82, 84Q/85A
  advantages/disadvantages, 80, 84Q/86A
  causes, 80
  cellular processes, 80-81, 84Q/85A:86A
  chemical mediators, 81, 82
  chronic, 82-83, 84Q/86-87A
  complement and, 41
  differentiation, 98-100
  exudate, 81, 84Q/85A, 120
  granulomatous, 83
  signs and symptoms, 80
Initiator, carcinogenesis, 121
Injury
  cellular response, 20

to cells, 30-31, 34Q/35A:36A
Integrins, 81
Interferons, 63, 121
Interleukins, 63, 65Q/67A, 121
Ischaemia, 34Q/36A, 121

K
Karyolysis, 31
Karyorrhexis, 31, 34Q/35A
Killer cells, 64
Kinin system, 40
Küppfer cells, 121

L
Laboratory investigations, 12-15, 16Q/17-18A
Learning skills, 1
Leukaemia, 24Q/26A
Leukotrienes, 70, 82
Lines of Zahn, 50, 52Q/53A
Lipids and atherosclerosis, 48, 52Q/53A
Lipofuscin, 22, 114
Liquefaction, 32, 33
Liver cells, 20, 22, 24Q/25A
Lymph nodes, 58, 59, 65Q/66A
Lymphocytes, 58-59
  inflammatory reactions, 80, 82
  see also B cells: T cells
Lymphoid follicles, 58
Lymphoid tissue, 58
Lymphoma, 121
Lysosomes, 80, 82, 121

M
Macrophages, 61, 63, 64, 80, 84Q/85-87A, 121
  atherosclerosis, 48
  epithelioid, 63, 83, 120
  inflammatory reactions, 81, 82
Major histocompatibility complex (MHC), 61, 63, 65Q/66A:67A, 72, 122
Malignant melanoma, 108
Margination, 121
Mast cells, 80
  degranulation, 70, 75Q/76A
  properties, 70
Mediator, 122
Melanin, 114, 116Q/118A
Membrane attack complex (MAC), 40, 41
Metalloproteinases, 91
Metaplasia, 21, 22-23, 24Q/25A, 98, 102Q/103-104A
Metastasis, 98-99, 107, 110Q/111A, 122
MHC, 61, 63, 65Q/66A:67A, 72, 122
Mitosis, 20
Molecular biology, diagnostic techniques, 14-15, 16Q/18A
Monoclonal antibodies, 13, 59
Monocytes, 80, 81-82, 122
Multiple myeloma, 59, 116Q/117A
Muscle cells, hypertrophic, 22
Myeloma, multiple see Multiple myeloma
Myocardial infarction, 51, 52Q/53A
Myocardium, 24Q/25A
  scarring, 92, 93Q/95A
Myofibroblast, 122

N
Necrosis, 32-33, 34Q/35A:36A, 122
Neoplasia, 22, 24Q/25A:26A, 98, 102Q/103A:104A
  apoptosis and, 31-32
  dysplasia and, 99-100
Neoplasms, 122
  benign, 106, 107
  growth, 106, 107
  malignant see Cancer
  nomenclature, 107-108

Neovascularisation, 90
Neural proteins, 14
Neutrophils, 80, 81-82, 84Q/87A, 122
Nitric oxide, 82
Northern blot analysis, 14-15

O
Occupational diseases, 4, 102Q/104A
Oedema, 81, 122
Onco-suppressor genes, 101
Oncogenes, 100-101, 122
  viral, 122
Oncoproteins, 122
Opsonisation, 40, 41, 44Q/45A:46A, 122
Osteoporosis, 24Q/26A

P
p53, 101
Pathogen, 122
Pathogenesis , 5, 6Q/9A
Perforin, 63
Periodic acid Schiff (PAS) stain, 13
Peyer's patches, 58
Phagocytosis, 31, 41, 44Q/46A, 80, 82, 122
Phagosome, 122
Pigments, accumulation in tissue, 114-115, 116Q/117A
Plasma cells, inflammatory reactions, 80, 82
Plasmin, 40, 42, 44Q/45A
Platelet activating factor (PAF), 82
Platelet-derived growth factor (PDGF), 48
Platelets, role in clotting, 41, 42, 44Q/45A
Polyclonal antibodies, 13
Polymerase chain reaction (PCR), 15, 16Q/18A
Prevalence of disease, 4, 6Q/8A:9A
Prognosis, 6Q/8A
Promoter, 122
Prostaglandins, 70, 82
Proto-oncogenes, 100-101, 122
Putrefaction, 122
Pyknosis, 31, 122

R
Regeneration, 20, 24Q/27A, 90, 93Q/95A, 122
Renal epithelial cells, 24Q/25A
Repair, 90, 93Q/95A, 122
Reticulin (Retic) stain, 13
Rhesus (Rh) blood group antigens, 70, 71
Rheumatoid disease, 72

S
Sarcoma, 107, 122
Scar/scarring, 91-92, 122
Screening, 6Q/8A
  cancer, 99, 100, 108, 110Q/112A
Serotonin, 82
Severe combined immunodeficiency disease (SCID), 73
Shock, 42-43, 44Q/45A
Signs, 12, 16Q/17A
Sjögren's syndrome, 72
Skin prick tests, 70, 75Q/76A
Skin wound healing, 90, 91, 93Q/95A
Southern blot analysis, 14-15, 59
Squamous cell carcinoma, markers, 16Q/17A
Stains, 12-13
Stem cell, 122-123
Streptococcal throat infection, 65Q/66-67A
Symptoms, 12, 16Q/17A
Systemic lupus erythematosus, 71, 72

T
T cells, 58, 61-63

cytotoxic, 62, 63, 64, 65Q/66A
delayed hypersensitivity, 62, 63
helper, 61, 62, 63, 64
receptors, 58, 59, 65Q/67A
subsets, 58, 61, 62
suppressor, 62, 63
Teratoma, 107, 123
Throat infection, streptococcal, 65Q/66-
    67A
Thrombin, 41-42
Thrombosis, 49-50, 51, 52Q/53A:54-55A,
    123
deep vein, 50, 52Q/53A
Thromboxane A2 (TXA2), 41, 42,
    44Q/45A, 48
Thymus, 58
Transient ischaemic attack, 50
Translocation, 123
Transplant rejection, 72-73, 75Q/77A
Transudate, 123
Tuberculin test, 71-72
Tuberculosis, 123
    immune response, 63
Tumour markers, 14, 16Q/17A, 108
Tumours *see* Cancer: Neoplasms

U
Ulcer, 123
    gastrointestinal, 91
Ultrastructural examination, 12
Urticaria, 70

V
Vacuoles, autophagic, 22
Vasodilatation, 81
Virchow's triad, 49

W
Western blot analysis, 14-15, 16Q/17A
Wound healing *see* Healing

Z
Ziehl Nielsen (ZN) stain, 13

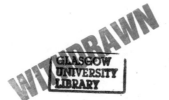